Massive, Muscular Arms

Scientifically Proven Strategies for Bigger Biceps, Triceps, and Forearms

David Barr

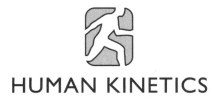

HUMAN KINETICS

Library of Congress Cataloging-in-Publication Data

Names: Barr, David, 1976- author.
Title: Massive, muscular arms : scientifically proven strategies for bigger biceps, triceps, and forearms / by David Barr.
Description: Champaign, IL : Human Kinetics, Inc., [2022] | Includes bibliographical references.
Identifiers: LCCN 2021005542 (print) | LCCN 2021005543 (ebook) | ISBN 9781718200876 (paperback) | ISBN 9781718200883 (epub) | ISBN 9781718200890 (pdf)
Subjects: LCSH: Arm exercises. | Strength training. | Exercise--Physiological aspects.
Classification: LCC GV508 .B37 2022 (print) | LCC GV508 (ebook) | DDC 613.7/1887--dc23
LC record available at https://lccn.loc.gov/2021005542
LC ebook record available at https://lccn.loc.gov/2021005543

ISBN: 978-1-7182-0087-6 (print)

Acquisitions Editor: Michael Mejia; **Developmental Editor:** Anne Hall; **Managing Editor:** Shawn Donnelly; **Copyeditor:** Janet Kiefer; **Permissions Manager:** Martha Gullo; **Senior Graphic Designer:** Joe Buck; **Cover Designer:** Keri Evans; **Cover Design Specialist:** Susan Rothermel Allen; **Photograph (cover):** zeljkosantrac / E+/ Getty Images; **Photographs (interior):** Adam Bratten/© Human Kinetics, unless otherwise noted; **Photo Asset Manager:** Laura Fitch; **Photo Production Specialist:** Amy M. Rose; **Photo Production Manager:** Jason Allen; **Senior Art Manager:** Kelly Hendren; **Illustrations:** © Human Kinetics, unless otherwise noted; **Printer:** The P.A. Hutchison Company

We thank Anytime Fitness in Colorado Springs, Colorado (Cheyenne Mountain), for assistance in providing the location for the photo shoot for this book.

Human Kinetics books are available at special discounts for bulk purchase. Special editions or book excerpts can also be created to specification. For details, contact the Special Sales Manager at Human Kinetics.

Printed in the United States of America

10 9 8 7 6 5 4 3 2 1

The paper in this book is certified under a sustainable forestry program.

Human Kinetics
1607 N. Market Street
Champaign, IL 61820
USA

United States and International
Website: **US.HumanKinetics.com**
Email: info@hkusa.com
Phone: 1-800-747-4457

Canada
Website: **Canada.HumanKinetics.com**
Email: info@hkcanada.com

E8214

Tell us what you think!
Human Kinetics would love to hear what we can do to improve the customer experience. Use this QR code to take our brief survey.

This work is dedicated to the dozens of individuals who have unknowingly contributed, from: UW, T Nation, M&F, EliteFTS, NSCA, ACSM, PPSC, and HK. Thank you for your patience and generosity in helping an Aspie kid as he fumbled his way through life in pursuit of performance optimization.

Contents

PART III   THE PROGRAMS   223

Exercise Finder

Introduction: Why Arms?

The legend of Eric began with his new position as head strength coach for a university soccer club. The team was not particularly talented or expected to do well in the upcoming season, but that didn't matter. This was still Eric's dream job. He had meticulously planned out every aspect of the team's training, from off-season all the way through an overly optimistic playoff schedule. Every detail seemed to be considered, until team captain Brian threw a wrench into the program.

"We need to train arms," was Brian's first response after looking at the off-season program. This surprising statement (*not* request) was coming from a respected soccer player who probably knew that there are a hundred other priorities to train for performance.

But this wasn't about physical performance. It was about psychological domination.

Brian was aware of the team's skill limits and knew that they needed a different edge. He explained to Eric that some of his teammates were more muscular than average, and they could use this to their advantage. The coach liked where the idea was headed and incorporated arm training into the end of lifting sessions twice per week.

The deceptively simple plan was for the team to warm up before the match with their shirts off. While none of the athletes were going to set the bodybuilding world on fire, they looked like Adonises compared to the pipe cleaner physiques of their competitors. The resulting warm-up drew gazes from fans and opposing teams alike, to the extent that one opposing coach could be heard shouting at his team to focus on the prematch drills.

Even once the jerseys were donned, the sleeves were rolled up to fully expose the impressive arm musculature of the team. This in-your-face tactic served as a constant reminder of what the opponent was about to contend with. The double-sided confidence boost and intimidation ploy worked beautifully, and on the field Brian and Eric's team routinely won physical matchups against now-hesitant rivals. This effect contributed to a few hard-fought and surprising victories over more highly skilled teams, which ultimately led to a very exciting playoff run. Although Eric joked that his preparation for playoffs was the difference maker, he gave most of the credit to Brian for having identified the power of the arms.

The anecdote about Eric is just one example of why so many are obsessed with these muscles. Consider that other than body modification and tattoos, your physique is the one thing that makes a statement about you as soon as you enter a room, before you even say a word. And it says *a lot*. People know what it means—dedication, intensity, attraction, and power.

Your arms are especially susceptible to this judgment, because they are a key part of the frame muscles—those that help you fill up a door frame and contribute to your overall silhouette. They are also the most visible of all body parts, which is obvious when considering how common T-shirts are. When you develop a set of muscular arms, don't be surprised if your wardrobe suddenly develops a lack of long sleeves in turn.

This instinctive drive for arm development is nothing new, as even the bodybuilders of the '60s and '70s obsessed over them. There was no shortage of awesome body parts for Arnold Schwarzenegger, but his arms are arguably the most famous. Their mere mention probably conjures images of one of his signature biceps poses—the right peak of which seemed to mimic the very Austrian Alps that he so proudly envisioned while training them.

But in spite of the early success of the golden age bodybuilders, training has evolved to a huge degree. Science has made the old-school thinking of pounding your biceps and triceps with excessive volume a thing of the past. In fact, that tradition may be effective for those who are chemically enhanced, but research has shown that excessive volume can hurt your gains (Benito et al. 2020).

Throughout this book we'll apply this science, so you can develop bigger arms by training smarter, not longer. We'll explore techniques to make your training safe, effective, *and* interesting; you might even find some of this to be fun! Best of all, you'll see the same principles I've successfully used with dozens of clients and athletes, to build your own set of dangerous "guns."

PART I

The Science

Biceps, Triceps, and Forearms: Know the Goal

Everyone wants to develop lean, muscular arms, but there's something different about you. The fact that you're spending the time and energy to read these words shows that you're willing to do more than most. You want more than the traditional information that's been floating around and regurgitated for the past 50 years. It's time to break out of the Iron Age and apply the following upgrades to optimize your physique.

Upgrade 1: By **reverse engineering** the goal, we are in a much better position to achieve it. In this case we'll start with the end in mind, by asking, "How does muscle grow?" Don't worry, you don't have to actually answer that. The heavy lifting has been done here for you, so not only will you be able to see the simplified answer, but you'll be able to apply it for optimal growth.

Upgrade 2: Another step beyond tradition lies in the form of **personalization**. Although you are encouraged to use the set, rep, and load schemes (etc.) presented, you have the potential to realize even faster results by personalizing each workout. This means that you'll see how, with experience, you'll be able to tailor your own training to each workout, each set, and even each rep. That's a level of customization that translates to optimized growth.

We'll come to apply these upgrades through the five key targets discussed in this book. There's no time to waste, so let's jump in by taking a very different look at anatomy and change the way you view traditional training.

KEY 1: ANATOMICALLY TARGETED TRAINING

We'll begin the processes of reverse engineering and personalization by first exploring anatomy. Naturally, this refers to your own body, but we'll also dissect the anatomy of your training. By understanding each, you'll see how they can be used to upgrade your arm development.

It might not seem intuitive, but the first key to arm development is being able to identify what it is that you're training. For example, just by understanding the anatomy of the arms, you can really focus on how to engage each muscle through different exercises and improve your overall results. You can also design a more effective workout plan by incorporating different movements that take full advantage of the variety of muscle-stimulating actions.

Anatomy Basics

After this introduction to arm anatomy, you may be quick to experience those benefits. From your very next workout, you will be able to play with different movements and different contractions, resulting in a better feel for the muscles you are trying to grow. With that in mind, let's jump into the first essential key toward your optimal gains.

Major Muscles and Bones

- The **humerus** is the large upper arm bone between the shoulder and forearm that we associate with the biceps and triceps muscles (figure 1.1*a*).
- The **biceps muscle** consists of two heads (*bi* = two; *cep* = head): the long head on the outside (lateral) and the short head on the inside (medial) (figure 1.1*a*).
- The **triceps muscle** consists of three heads: the long, medial, and lateral (figure 1.1*b*).
- The bones of the forearm are the **radius** on the outside (lateral) and **ulna** (medial) when your palm is turned up.
- The shoulder blade is called the **scapula** and serves as an attachment point for both the biceps and triceps.

Primary Functions

The main function of the biceps is elbow flexion (as you do in biceps curls), and the main function of the triceps is to straighten the elbow, which is known as extension. These opposing muscle actions are the reason the biceps and triceps are often identified as **antagonist muscles**.

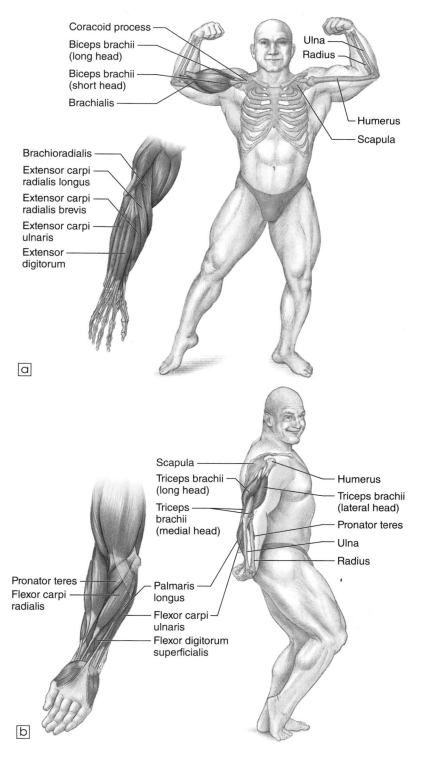

Coracoid process
Biceps brachii (long head)
Biceps brachii (short head)
Brachialis
Ulna
Radius
Humerus
Scapula

Brachioradialis
Extensor carpi radialis longus
Extensor carpi radialis brevis
Extensor carpi ulnaris
Extensor digitorum

a

Scapula
Triceps brachii (long head)
Triceps brachii (medial head)
Humerus
Triceps brachii (lateral head)
Pronator teres
Ulna
Radius

Pronator teres
Flexor carpi radialis
Palmaris longus
Flexor carpi ulnaris
Flexor digitorum superficialis

b

Figure 1.1   (*a*) The humerus, biceps, and wrist extensors; (*b*) the triceps and wrist flexors.

Each of the muscles cross both the shoulder and elbow joint. For this reason, they are said to be *biarticular*. At first this may seem like insignificant trivia, but you'll soon see that it will have a strong impact on how you train these muscle groups.

Secondary Functions

Because they cross the shoulder, the biceps also cause shoulder **flexion**. This movement can be described as the humerus moving from vertical at your side, to horizontal in front of the body, and then continuing to end vertically overhead. The barbell front raise (figure 1.2) is one common example of this type of motion, and the overhead triceps press (figure 1.3) shows the maximally flexed end range of motion.

Based on the way the biceps insert onto the forearm bones, they also perform an action called **supination**. This refers to turning the palm up. A common cue to remember supination is to think of the palm turning up to hold soup in your hand (the pronunciation of supination begins with *soup*). You may even hear a personal trainer cueing a client with the reminder of "pinky up" during a set of biceps curls (figure 1.4). The opposite movement (turning the palm down) is called **pronation**. For example, when you perform triceps push-downs with a straight bar, your wrists are pronated (figure 1.5).

Like the biceps, the triceps also crosses the shoulder joint and performs the opposite movement, called **shoulder extension**. You probably experience this type of contraction most often during your back training, because rowing movements (figure 1.6) are great examples of shoulder extension.

Essential Application

Changing both the shoulder (Barakat et al. 2019) and wrist position (Kleiber et al. 2015) can affect arm muscle activation. Employing a variety of muscle-specific exercises that use these different joint positions will help you to **recruit** as much of the muscle as possible for maximal growth. This maximal recruitment strategy is the essence of the key target, anatomically targeted training.

Other Muscles

Muscles that assist the biceps in elbow flexion are the **brachialis**, which is large but hidden underneath the biceps, and the **brachioradialis**, which looks more like a forearm muscle. The brachialis should not be neglected, because it adds overall muscle mass to the arm, but it is impossible to isolate during training. For this reason, we'll usually refer to the elbow flexor group collectively as biceps.

We'll also refer to the muscles that pull your wrist toward your body (when the palm is up) as **wrist flexors**. Collectively, the muscles that perform that opposite action are the **wrist extensors** (see figures 1.1*a* and 1.1*b*).

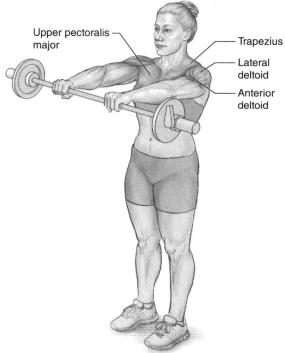

Upper pectoralis major

Trapezius

Lateral deltoid

Anterior deltoid

Figure 1.2 Barbell front raise.

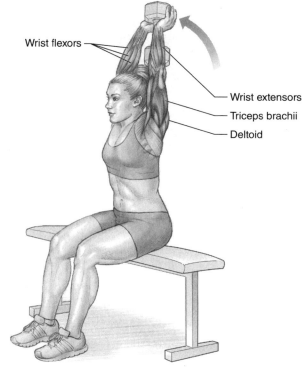

Wrist flexors

Wrist extensors

Triceps brachii

Deltoid

Figure 1.3 Triceps press.

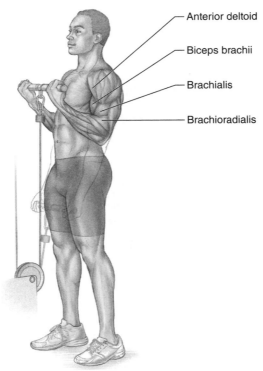

Anterior deltoid

Biceps brachii

Brachialis

Brachioradialis

Figure 1.4 Cable curl.

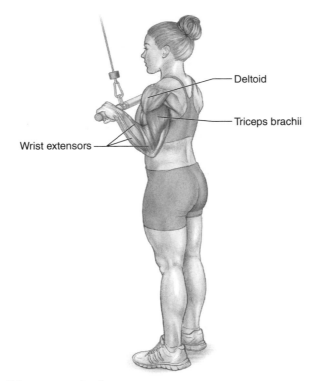

Deltoid

Triceps brachii

Wrist extensors

Figure 1.5 Triceps push-down.

SideBarr

You may see or hear the muscles of the arm occasionally called biceps brachii and triceps brachii. This is to distinguish these arm muscles from the biceps femoris and triceps surae muscles that we have in our legs. For the purposes of this book, we'll only consider the arm (brachial) versions of these muscles.

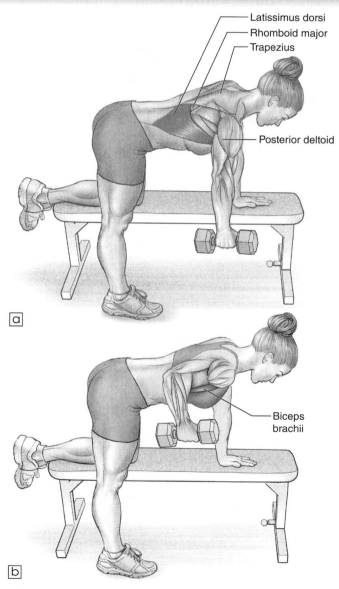

Figure 1.6 Dumbbell row (*a*) start position; (*b*) finish position.

ANATOMY OF A REP

Along with using your physical anatomy, we'll take your training to the next level by dissecting the applied anatomy of your workout. This begins with the three types of muscle contraction that can translate into phases of your reps.

Concentric contractions refer to the shortening of the muscle, and they happen when your muscle exerts more force than that of the load acting against it. A common example is starting at the bottom of a biceps curl and flexing the elbow to peak contraction. This is also referred to as the concentric phase of the rep and is illustrated in figure 1.7 as the solid horizontal line.

If you were to hold this top position of the curl, your biceps are still contracting to resist the load, even though it is not moving. This type of contraction, in which the muscle does not shorten or lengthen, is an **isometric** (*iso* = same, *metric* = length measurement) **contraction**. It is represented by the center vertical line (figure 1.7). Even if they are incredibly brief, there is still an isometric contraction as you transition between the other two phases of your rep (from concentric to eccentric and vice versa). These are occasionally called static contractions, and they are the result of your muscle exerting force equal to that acting against it.

Isometric contractions also happen when you maintain muscle tension at the bottom of the movement, or anytime the muscle contracts to produce force but does not change length. In fact, unless you're in an all-out sprint as you read these words, you have dozens of muscles contracting isometrically (to resist gravity) right now! Also note that your wrist flexors and extensors are isometrically contracted throughout the entire set of biceps curls to stabilize the wrist.

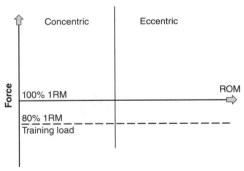

Figure 1.7 Force output during a single repetition. The vertical axis represents the amount of force. The horizontal axis represents the change in range of motion (ROM) as a repetition is performed, starting with the concentric movement and progressing to the eccentric movement. The solid horizontal line occurs at the level of maximal force that can be overcome for a single repetition (one rep maximum; 100 percent 1RM). The force exerted by an 80 percent 1RM training load is shown as the horizontal dashed line.

The potential benefits of isometric contractions also warrant your consideration. Although not overlooked as often as eccentric contractions, many people still ignore the important potential of isometric holds. This common knowledge gap means that you can gain another advantage by using the tools described in this book. In fact, you'll soon see different ways to use this contraction as a versatile weapon to boost your gains.

The controlled descent of the biceps curl (returning to starting position) involves the active lengthening of the muscle, known as an **eccentric contraction** (also known as a negative). As you might expect, this is also called the eccentric phase of the rep.

Other essential components of repetition anatomy relate to the exercise movement and the relative load. The **range of motion (ROM)** is the degree of movement that happens throughout an exercise, which is typically limited by the mobility of the joint. For example, barbell biceps curls begin with the elbows maximally extended and end when the elbows cannot flex further. That description applies to the concentric portion of the movement, and most exercises reverse direction for the same ROM during the eccentric portion.

The maximum load that you can overcome with good form for a single rep is your **1-repetition maximum (1RM)** for that exercise, which is often used as a benchmark for subsequent training loads. For example, if you can curl 100 pounds (45 kg) only once before your form breaks down, this is your 1RM. You'll load each exercise with a reduced percentage of this in order to perform multiple consecutive reps. For example, 80 percent of your 1RM would be 80 lb (36 kg), which could serve as your training load.

The barbell biceps curl serves as our walkthrough of the figures, because this exercise starts at the bottom position (with elbows fully extended) and the concentric contraction (elbow flexion). When you reach maximal flexion, there is a brief pause (isometric contraction), represented by the middle vertical line. The eccentric contraction follows, as you descend to starting position to perform another rep.

We all tend to get a little lazy during the eccentric part of the rep, but you'll have better results if you do not think of the negative as muscle relaxation—it is an active muscle contraction and should be treated that way.

We tend to focus on the concentric phase because we are weaker during this portion of a rep (figure 1.8), and as a result, we have to expend more energy and effort during each. This often means that the eccentric portion is a throwaway, to be treated like a brief rest before the next "real" effort of the concentric portion. Just observe someone as they perform a hard set of dumbbell presses to fatigue and watch what happens after they complete that final brutal concentric movement; you can bet money on the fact that they'll effectively drop the load, only controlling the momentum enough to avoid injury as the iron comes to a stop on their thighs or the ground.

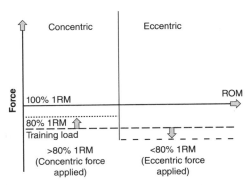

Figure 1.8 Force output during one full repetition. The force required during the concentric phase is greater than the load, and that of the eccentric phase is less than the load. These force differences are shown relative to an example of an 80 percent 1RM load with upward and downward arrows, respectively.

This instinct is so common because the human body wants to be efficient (read: lazy) and preserve energy for survival. Combine this with the fact that we're used to concentrically overcoming gravity, not only in training, but with every step we've ever taken. This means that we have years of experience, naturally working harder to fight gravity concentrically and taking breaks during each subsequent eccentric phase. It is important for your growth that this survival-based efficiency doesn't translate into training-day complacency.

We can begin to fully appreciate our untapped potential when comparing our training loads with the actual amount of force we're capable of producing. This begins with a visual representation to illustrate that we're capable of producing relatively high forces during common movements, which are shown as our natural **force potential** (figure 1.9).

We can't feel this difference when we're training, so it's important to note the size of the vertical arrows shown in figure 1.10. These represent the **force deficit**, which is the difference between our force potential and actual forces produced during training. Note that the deficit is much greater for eccentric contractions, because we are much stronger during this phase and yet must produce less eccentric force during training. This extends the deficit in both directions, which is called the **eccentric paradox**.

Another training secret is that we are much stronger eccentrically (as the muscle lengthens under load) and we can take advantage of this force potential for even better results. In upcoming chapters, you will see how eccentric movements can be used in two completely different ways to accelerate your strength and muscle growth, and how they might even reduce injury risk.

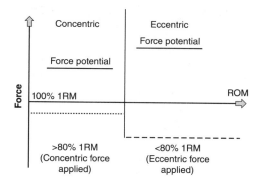

Figure 1.9 Force potential differences over the course of a single repetition. Horizontal lines above the 100 percent 1RM line show the maximal amount of force that the muscle can produce, which is called force potential.

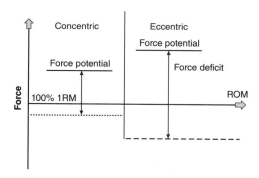

Figure 1.10 Force deficit and the eccentric paradox. The difference between force potential and actual force exerted during a repetition is the force deficit which is represented by the vertical double ended arrows. A longer vertical arrow during the eccentric phase illustrates the enormous force deficit during this phase. The fact that we are much stronger eccentrically (i.e., have higher force potential) but exert less force during this part of the repetition is called the eccentric paradox.

SHATTERING BARRIERS

Now that we've seen the magnitude of the limits, you should know what causes them, so you can ultimately crush them and see them driven before you. For this reason, we'll apply reverse engineering to our reps and sets, for the final component of your anatomically targeted training. As a reminder, we do this so we can break through these self-imposed barriers and come to improve our workouts and subsequent arm development. Figure 1.11 illustrates how we restrict our training loads due to specific parts of our ROM and the need to perform multiple consecutive contractions.

The **concentric constraint (con-con)** illustrates the fact that we immediately limit the load of every training set to our concentric portion of the rep. Note that we do not simply ignore the stronger eccentric portion; we actually have to exert even less force during this phase, which we've seen is the eccentric paradox. We'll deal with this important concept in upcoming chapters, but for now will stay focused on traditional training loads.

After limiting our load to the weakest half of the full rep, we are further bound by our **concentric range of motion** (**con-ROM;** not to be confused with the similar sounding genre of film). This component is especially important because it is the portion of the full concentric ROM where we have the greatest difference between the force we need to overcome and our force potential. This restrictive part of the ROM is commonly called the **sticking point** of an exercise, and it establishes the traditional holy grail of loading, the 1RM. It's worth emphasizing that for traditional training, *the greatest measure of strength is established by the weakest part of the ROM, from the weakest part of the rep.*

Although the external load itself does not change during a movement (e.g., a 10lb dumbbell doesn't change during a curl), the force required by the muscle to overcome that load can change, due to mechanical advantages across the joint. The difference between the minimum and maximum required force production across an ROM is called the **force delta**, and can be an important consideration for optimizing your muscle development.

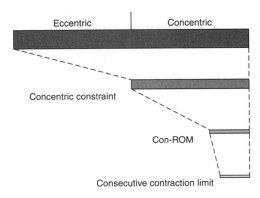

Figure 1.11   A simplified representation of the relative proportion of self-imposed limits common with traditional resistance training.

A dumbbell lateral raise provides a great example of a changing resistance throughout the ROM. As you abduct the arm to parallel (with the ground), the resistance progressively increases due to the leverage across the shoulder joint (figures 1.12*a* and 1.12*b*). In this extreme scenario, there is effectively zero load at the bottom of the movement (with your arms hanging at your sides), compared with maximal load at the end of the concentric portion.

Practically speaking, force delta is a primary determining factor for how much load you use during a set. It becomes particularly noteworthy when there is a large change in resistance across the ROM. Because the load of the exercise is selected based on the ROM with the greatest need for force production (i.e. at the sticking point), a large force delta would mean that the entire training load is limited by that small part of the total exercise ROM. As a result, this load would only serve as a maximally effective stimulus to the muscle across that relatively small portion of the full movement.

An **extreme force delta** happens during exercises that have very high relative loading at one end of the ROM, and effectively zero load at the other. Examples of common exercises with an extreme force delta include dumbbell lateral raises, dumbbell pec flys, and preacher curls. This doesn't mean that you need to avoid these exercises. You should just be aware of their limits and include exercises that anatomically target the muscle across other parts of the ROM.

Returning to the dumbbell lateral raise example, you may experience the desired muscle tension only during the final degrees of the ROM (at the end of the concentric movement). The first third of the exercise provides

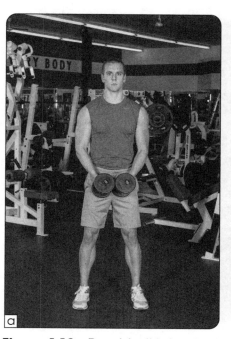 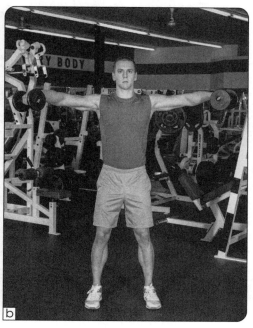

Figure 1.12 Dumbbell lateral raise.

negligible resistance, which translates to minimal stimulus for the working muscle. To compensate you might also include cable lateral raises in your program (figures 1.13*a* and 1.13*b*), which target the shoulder at the bottom of the movement. The strategy of using different exercises to stimulate a muscle across a broader ROM has been aptly described to me as **full-range strength** by personal training educator Nick Tumminello. You'll come to see how these concepts are used to maximize your arm development as we continue to apply them in upcoming chapters (3, 5, and 7).

In order to perform consecutive full ROM contractions, which we know as a set, the load must be further reduced from the con-ROM. The **consecutive contraction limit** is typically expressed as a percentage of 1RM (figure 1.11 uses 80 percent as an example).

In summary, figure 1.11 provides a simple visual representation of some limits we impose on ourselves during traditional training. The relative size of the final bar compared to the larger top bar is meant to offer a figurative but clear perspective for our untapped potential.

It is important that this information is not viewed as negative, or that it suggests that traditional training is dispensable. Rather, it is simply intended to offer a look at some of the current limits to our muscle stimuli. Once this perspective is achieved, we are free to break these barriers and upgrade the stimuli using a rational approach to training.

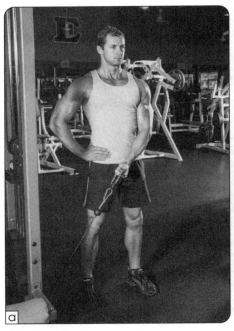
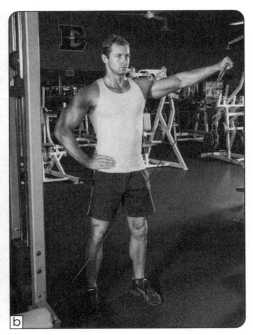

Figure 1.13   Cable lateral raise.

SideBarr

In contrast to convenient or concise, you may conclude that any consideration to convey conjoined concepts as *con-con-con-ROM-con-con-lim* is convincingly convoluted, if not contemptuous.

WRAP-UP

This section provided a sneak preview of the key targets that you'll use to optimize your arm development. These begin by reverse engineering how your muscle grows and the methods used to cause this effect. By introducing personalization into your training, you'll quickly be able to improve each workout and the physical results that follow.

These concepts were applied through the key to anatomically targeted training. By optimizing your personal anatomy, as well as that of your reps, you'll be ahead of the game when it comes to muscle development.

The Science Says . . . : A Smarter Way to Train

With the importance of targeted anatomy now firmly established, let's explore the next key target. If anatomy is the *what*, then this is the start of the *how*. We discussed key 1 in the first chapter; we'll continue with keys 2 through 4 in this chapter.

KEY 2: TARGETED TRAINING PARAMETERS

You may find it helpful if we develop this key, starting with traditional training concepts. As we progress throughout the book, we'll continually add to these techniques, providing you with more weapons in your training arsenal. This progressive addition will ensure that the concepts are understood first, which will help to facilitate your application and ultimately, your arm development.

The American College of Sports Medicine (ACSM) is a leading health and fitness organization that puts out simple but thoroughly researched exercise guidelines. One of its most accessible recommendations describes exercise programming variables: frequency, intensity, time, type, volume, and progression (American College of Sports Medicine 2021, 142).

Because you're predominantly resistance-exercise focused, this concept has been adapted to not only keep it simple but also to increase its precision and effectiveness. These **targeted training parameters** are your second key to dominating your arm training (see table 2.2 on page 23).

Frequency

This programming variable refers to how often you train each muscle group. Although frequency can be a basic component of your program, it takes on a layer of complexity when optimizing arm training. Your arms are also used in other upper body movements. Anytime you're holding a load, they can still take a beating, even if you're not training them directly. In fact, research has shown that stimulating the arms via multijoint (e.g., seated row) versus isolated single-joint (e.g., biceps curl) movements will cause different levels of biceps stress and will subsequently affect recovery adaptation times (Soares et al. 2015).

Common examples of this carryover effect to the arms include rowing movements for the back and overhead pressing for the shoulders. This indirect stimulation will factor into the frequency of direct arm training days as well as other workouts that may affect your arm development.

Intensity

Intensity refers to the load that is used for the working set and is expressed as a percent of **1-repetition maximum (1RM)**. For example, if you can curl a maximum of 100 pounds (45 kg) only once with good form, that load is your 1RM. To apply this equation to your working set, you could use a load intensity of 65 pounds (29 kg) or 65 percent 1RM, for example.

In a more subjective application, intensity can be used to describe the level of effort you put into each working set. Continuing with the previous example, if you can curl your 65 percent 1RM 10 times before failing, a very hard intensity level could mean that you perform seven or eight reps, stopping just short of muscular failure.

This measure is intentionally subjective because your perceived effort varies not only from day to day, but from set to set. In this way, you can be incredibly specific about your level of intensity in real time. This is the first important step toward personalizing your workouts.

You can quantify your degree of effort using a **rating of perceived exertion (RPE)** scale (see table 2.1). Although there are different RPE scales, we'll stick with the 10-point scale because of its simplicity. The number is used to establish your relative effort during the hardest part of the exercise and to provide a personalized level of intensity.

Time Under Tension

Although *time* can refer to the duration of a lifting session (which is usually 40-90 minutes), it's more effective for you to think of this as a duration of each set. This is otherwise known as **time under tension (TUT)**, and it reflects how long a muscle is working under load.

Table 2.1   10-Point RPE Scale

Rating	Perceived exertion
1	Nothing at all (lying down)
2	Extremely little
3	Very easy
4	Easy (could do this all day)
5	Moderate
6	Somewhat hard (starting to feel it)
7	Hard
8	Very hard (making an effort to keep up)
9	Very very hard
10	Maximum effort (can't go any further)

Reprinted by permission from NSCA, "Aerobic Endurance Training Program Design," by P. Hagerman. in *NSCA's Essentials of Personal Training,* 2nd ed., edited by J.W. Coburn and M.H. Malek (Champaign, IL: Human Kinetics, 2012), 395.

TUT is used predominantly to indicate that the muscle should be exposed to tension for relatively longer durations in order to stimulate **hypertrophy** (also known as [aka] muscle growth). As an example, strength-focused training requires the use of heavy loads but minimal accumulation of fatigue. To achieve this, low TUT sets are performed using few concentric reps and long rest periods between those sets. We'll expand upon this with the parameter of tempo, shortly. TUT will be explored further in key target 4 (precision microtargeting) later in this chapter.

Type

Type describes the kind of equipment and its intended purpose for your program. For your resistance training focus, we'll use this parameter to identify the specific type of implement. Examples include dumbbells, barbells, kettlebells, selectorized machines, cables, elastic, suspension, body weight, and medicine balls. Each type has its own set of restrictions which helps to illustrate the need for training variety. Common examples of these limits include

- body-weight training, during which the load is limited;
- elastic resistance, which needs a secure anchor point; and
- barbell movements, which are bound by the limits of gravity and subsequent momentum.

Note that in spite of the wide variety of methods, nearly all the types use gravity as the resistance. We'll play with a broad range of resistances to keep your training interesting and accelerate growth.

Tempo

The **tempo** relates to how quickly you perform each of the four parts of a repetition: eccentric, maximal lengthened position, concentric, and peak contraction. Each section is numerically expressed in seconds.

For example, a set with a 4/1/2/1 tempo indicates a four-second eccentric part followed by a one-second pause, then a two-second concentric part before a one-second peak contraction pause. The next rep starts over with the four-second eccentric part.

Some programs might describe tempo using only three numbers, with the only difference being the omission of the peak contraction duration (i.e., the final number). In this case, the aforementioned example would then look like 4/1/2.

Tempo is one of the most overlooked components of any training program. It is commonly used only to indicate slower reps or very fast reps (in which case a 0 is used for the concentric part), but it is an important parameter for high-performance resistance training that will help you to keep your attention focused throughout each part of the rep. Key 4 (discussed later in this chapter) and key 5 (discussed in the next chapter) will show you why this focus is important for achieving your biggest gains. As a universal application, a tempo of 2/0/1/0 can be used when this parameter is not explicitly provided.

You can calculate the TUT of a set by multiplying the total tempo of one rep by the number of reps. First add the total number of seconds for one rep's tempo, and then multiply that number by the number of reps in each set.

Example: 2/0/1/0 [3 seconds for each rep] × 10 reps = 30-second TUT

Volume

Although it is often simplified as a product of sets, reps, and load, training volume is far more complicated than is often appreciated (Schoenfeld et al. 2019). Training parameters such as contraction type and rep range of motion (ROM) affect the amount of growth stimulus on the muscle but are typically left out of volume calculations. For the sake of simplicity and personalization, we'll define each training parameter where necessary rather than offer a prescribed complex training volume.

A generalization is that traditional periodization recommends an inverse relationship between training volume and intensity, which means that as one component goes up, the other decreases. For our purposes, this concept will be generally adapted so that the more intense the training, the less of it you'll do (and vice versa).

Progression

This strategic principle considers how the other training variables change over the course of weeks or months, in order to keep your muscle stimulated for adaptation. As muscle adapts, it becomes more resistant to change, so you need **progression** to mix up the workouts and keep the muscle adapting to different stresses. You might see this concept called the muscle confusion principle.

Bonus

The other important feature of progression is to keep your head in the game. No one wants to do the same thing week after week, so mix it up and keep it fun!

Table 2.2 Summary of Training Variables

Training variable	Definition
Frequency	How often
Intensity	How hard
Time (under tension)	How long (set)
Type	Resistance
Tempo	How long (each of the four parts of a rep)
Volume	How much
Progression	How to change

KEY 3: ADAPTIVE TARGETING

The next key target begins with a question of *why*? More specifically, *why do you lift?*

You probably don't think of why you lift beyond working out to increase muscle size and strength, which is totally fine. But as with every other key, we'll reverse engineer the concept to give you a better understanding of the fundamentals and then build toward advanced application. When we're done, you'll not only have the tools to improve your gains, but you'll be able to avoid the common mistakes that hold back so many others.

Consider that right now, your body is at a comfortable and balanced set point known as **homeostasis**. By disrupting this physiological state, your body will work to first restore stability and then adapt by becoming more resistant to subsequent disruptions. This is what you do with resistance training.

Some have described the stress and adaptation process as tearing down muscle with the lifting session, so that your body rebuilds it bigger and stronger than before. An even more scientifically accurate version states that you impose stresses on the muscle that stimulate it to adapt, which you experience in the form of muscle growth, strength, power, and so on.

It sounds strange right? We usually think of stress as a bad thing. But we exercise to intentionally induce overload stress on the muscle. The good news is that exercise provides positive stresses, in contrast to the emotional stresses that we usually refer to in a negative way. With training, we're using positive stress to stimulate long-term adaptation, so it's probably better if we think of exercise stress as a **stress stimulus**.

Metarecovery

Before we go too much further, we need to make an important distinction. Because it is one of the most misunderstood concepts in training, it's essential to note that we have different types of recovery, based on when they occur and how long they last.

In spite of their differences, the basic definition is the same for each: **recovery** is simply a return to where you started before some kind of deficit. Whether it's return to normal function after a broken arm, or rehydrating after a long hot run, recovery is all about getting back to zero.

One type you're no doubt familiar with is the **intermediate recovery** period that happens within the minutes and early hours after a lift. Intermediate recovery is best characterized by postworkout nutritional interventions such as rehydration, or replenishing muscle glycogen by eating carbohydrates. Ultimately, the goal of this brief period matches the very definition of recovery, which is merely a return to where you started, but not moving beyond.

Sneak Preview

In chapter 8 we'll go over some intermediate recovery techniques that should make your life easier and may even potentiate your long-term recovery adaptation.

Chain Reaction

We're talking about how to achieve bigger and faster gains, which are the result of a second type of recovery: **long-term recovery adaptation**. In contrast to intermediate recovery, long-term recovery adaptation happens over the course of several days following your workout and ends with an adaptive response (e.g., the muscle responds to the initial training stress by adapting, which we experience as bigger and tougher muscle).

For example, if muscle growth is initiated by the workout stress stimulus and ends with your desired adaptation of the muscle (i.e., hypertrophy), then you already have the first and final components of the entire process (see table 2.3). The workout (phase 1) begins a physiological chain reaction in your muscle that cascades through three more phases (described shortly) in the days that follow, ultimately leaving you with the growth and strength that you're after.

What may be counterintuitive is that the muscle soreness, fatigue, and the like, that you often experience a day or two *after* a workout is just the result your body's natural **stress response** (phase 2; aka preadaptation phase). It may not feel like it, but this response is actually an important part of the process because it sets up your subsequent **long-term recovery** and **adaptation** phases (phases 3 and 4, respectively). This means that soreness after a workout can be thought of as a good thing, and not something you should try to get rid of. Note that this soreness differs from pain experienced *during* a workout, either by acidity (commonly experienced as a burning sensation) or acute injury.

Table 2.3 Long-Term Recovery Adaptation in Four Phases

Phase	Recovery or adaptation response
1—Stress stimulus	Happens by overloading the muscle during your workout and starts the entire cascade.
2—Stress response	Occurs in the hours and days following the workout in order to prepare the muscle for adaptation. It is the time when your body clears away damaged tissue through the necessary process of inflammation, which you may temporarily experience as delayed-onset muscle soreness, swelling, decreased strength, or the like.
3—Recovery (long term)	The phase during which your body begins to rebuild the damaged tissue and get back to where you started.
4—Adaptation	Going beyond where you started. This is where you get bigger, faster, and stronger. Ultimately, this is what you're after.

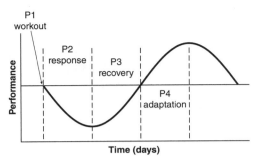

Figure 2.1   The Selye curve representing the four phases of long-term recovery adaptation. The workout (P1) is the stress stimulus that begins the series of recovery adaptation processes. The stress response (P2) is a natural preparatory phase that may be experienced as soreness. Recovery (P3) ends with a return to baseline performance. P4 is the desired adaptation phase, resulting in improved performance.

This entire process can be visually described by tracking performance over time, which results in a curved line known as the **Selye recovery adaptation curve** (figure 2.1). *Performance* is a general term, but let's think of it as strength in this example, and track what happens to you after a workout using the graph.

Strength naturally decreases a little over the early hours or days (P2; phase 2) after resistance training, which you may experience as mild muscle fatigue. Recall that this slight drop in strength is an organic part of the chain, which happens as the body clears away damaged tissue and ultimately sets up for adaptation.

The phase 2 stress response is followed by strength recovery (P3; phase 3) at the end of which you are back to where you started before the lift (i.e., zero deficit, zero gain). Lastly, several days after the process began, your body adapts, which you experience as a strength increase (P4; phase 4).

This four-phase cycle happens every time you lift and illustrates how you can get better after each workout. You can tie in the principle of progression by training again at the peak of the adaptation phase to restimulate the entire cycle using your newfound strength. You'll see how to optimize progression in upcoming sections.

Hypertrophy Note

Although muscle doesn't get smaller in phase 2, these general stimulus-response-recovery adaptation principles apply for hypertrophy training.

Proportionality Principle

Even if you haven't directly experienced it, you may intuitively know that the bigger the lift, the bigger the gains. In general terms, the greater the volume, or the harder the workout, the greater result (figure 2.2).* This harder workout might come with more soreness and a longer recovery period, but the resulting growth makes the pain worthwhile. This applied concept illustrates the **proportionality principle**.

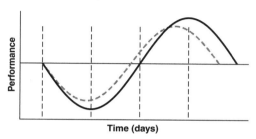

Figure 2.2 The recovery adaptation curve as a result of a more intense or higher volume workout (black) contrasted with an average workout (gray dashed curve). The four phases of the new curve (vertical dashed lines) illustrate changes from the original workout. Note that although performance is initially decreased to a greater degree, the adaptive response is proportionally larger.

Proportionality is also maintained with lighter workouts, which cause less of a stress stimulus and subsequently a smaller adaptive response (figure 2.3).

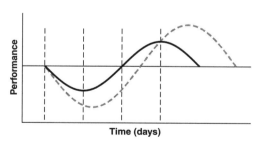

Figure 2.3 The recovery adaptation curve as a result of a light workout (black) contrasted with an average workout (gray dashed curve). The four phases of the new curve (vertical dashed lines) illustrate changes from the original workout. Note that although the return to baseline performance (i.e., recovery) happens faster, the adaptive response is proportionally smaller.

*You can easily go off the rails with too much volume and intensity, but by applying the guidelines provided in this book, the truism will hold.

SideBarr

There's a lot going on here so it may be helpful to solidify the concepts with the following rhyme: If more growth is desired, it becomes more required: make muscle more tired.

Although it's counterintuitive to want to induce muscle fatigue, this rhyme connects several concepts, including that of introducing a stimulus to cause adaptation.

More specifically, tired muscle represents two elements, beginning with the acute stress stimulus induced by the workout (P1). It also represents the preadaptation phase (P2), during which a delayed performance decrease occurs. Further, these necessary elements help to set up the desired adaptation. Lastly, the proportionality principle is represented by the idea that more stress stimulus results in more growth.

Reductive clue: If you want to play a scientist or meathead version of *The Da Vinci Code*, there's a hidden concept within this rhyme revealed shortly.

Applied Interventions

Your applied understanding of recovery interventions is about to put you way ahead of the pack, and we'll use the properties represented by the Selye curve to make it happen. Consider that this waveform is incredibly common in nature and used to represent patterns like those made by waves of light and sound, your heartbeat, or ripples in a pond, to name a few. By translating the impact of our workouts and subsequent interventions via changes in the curve, we can get a visual sense of what's happening in the body and how to optimize it.

For example, if recovery time and time to peak adaptation are decreased (i.e., happen faster), this is reflected on the curve as a shortened wavelength (see figure 2.3). This relative shortening is best described using a term derived from astrophysics, known as **blue shifting** (in reference to a relative increase in the frequency of light waves, as they shift toward the blue end of the visible spectrum). The act of blue shifting (i.e., reducing our recovery adaptation times) can easily be achieved by decreasing our relative training intensity or introducing specific recovery techniques. It may help you to remember this applied concept by thinking that

blue shifting blunts changes.

The opposite effect of **red shifting** comes with longer recovery and adaptation times, which is shown graphically by a longer wavelength (see figure 2.2). This relative change is typically desired, because the overall size of the curve is larger, which also means a greater adaptive response (aka bigger gains).

If you recall, that there's a hidden message embedded within the rhyme in the SideBarr, it will help you to remember the concepts of stress stimulus, stress response and the associated <u>red</u> shift (e.g., bigger initial deficit causes bigger adaptation). The hidden message is

if more growth is desi<u>red</u>, it becomes more requi<u>red</u>: make muscle more ti<u>red</u>.

These concepts are essential to understand because of the unintentionally blunted results caused by the gross misunderstanding of the words like inflammation, stress, and most importantly, recovery. Without the understanding of the four-phase concept, far too many people use recovery methods to get rid of soreness, decrease inflammation, or blindly accelerate recovery. Unfortunately, in doing so they often disrupt phase 2, preadaptation, short-circuit the entire chain, and ultimately hurt their gains. Common examples of these interventions include pain reliever anti-inflammatory drugs (e.g., NSAIDS, including aspirin), antioxidant supplements (e.g., high-dose vitamin C), and icing (i.e., decreasing muscle temperature to reduce inflammation).

The result of using these blue shifting techniques cause what is known as **destructive recovery** or **sacrificial recovery**. They destroy the stress response, thereby sacrificing adaptation, in order to minimize recovery time. So even if the workout (stress stimulus) is of high volume or very intense, artificially blunting the body's natural phase 2 response with common destructive recovery methods (during that phase) can effectively trick your muscle into adapting proportionally to a lighter workout.

For example, imagine a situation in which you crush a high-intensity workout with the intent to cause bigger gains (a red shift, illustrated in figure 2.2). If, after the workout, you were to use recovery techniques with the intent of decreasing soreness and inflammation, you'll decrease the size of the phase 2 response. Although it might temporarily feel better, this blunting of phase 2 causes a proportional decrease in phase 3 and then phase 4 (figure 2.3). This resulting blunted (i.e., blue shifted) curve is illustrated in figure 2.4.

In this sacrificial recovery scenario, you might experience less soreness and recover faster, but you've also wasted the effort of a hard workout by shooting yourself in the foot (i.e., you blunt your adaptative response, aka hurt your gains). If you had wanted to experience minimal soreness and a faster return to baseline performance, you could have replaced your high-intensity workout with a light day.

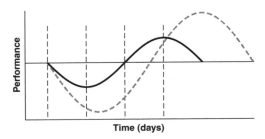

Figure 2.4 The natural recovery adaptation curve following a high-intensity workout (gray dashed curve) contrasted with the hypothetical result of having used inappropriate recovery interventions (black) during phase 2 following that same workout. The four phases of the new curve (vertical dashed lines) illustrate differences from the high-intensity workout. Note that although the return to baseline performance (i.e., recovery) happens faster due to the interventions, the adaptive response has been greatly decreased.

Lastly, you might recognize that your fellow lifters often confuse recovery for adaptation. Remember that recovery is about getting back to zero, but not going beyond. Although it is an important part of this chain, long-term recovery is *not* the end goal.

Hypertrophy Note

If you're looking to get better (bigger, stronger, faster, etc.), then it's critical to remember that your ultimate goal is *adaptation*.

KEY 4: PRECISION MICROTARGETING

We can build off keys 2 and 3 by advancing to the concepts of targeted growth and precise training specificity. This was a lesson I had to learn the hard way, beginning with my initial strength and conditioning experience.

Several years ago, I thought that I knew most of what there was to know about lifting. I had read several training books, studied anatomy, and applied what I had learned. So, I felt comfortable in saying "yes" when asked to work with college athletes and show them the ropes.

But I was dead wrong.

This was immediately clear as I watched the basketball team train their abs and core. Although I was aware of seemingly dozens of core and abdominal exercises, these athletes were training using an elongated torso, with one leg fully straight and the other bent. The confusion on my face must have been evident because the strength coach explained that this movement was used due to the occasional single leg nature of the sport, along with the tall position that the players often found themselves in.

Before I could fully wrap my head around this concept, I was humbled and surprised again by observing the squash athletes train. Their sport is executed in a low, almost hunched over stance, so all their exercises were performed with a similar body position. The real mind-blowing connection happened because this was in direct contrast to what I had just seen with the basketball athletes.

These initial experiences helped me to gain an appreciation for the vast amount of knowledge available (and a lot of humility), but also for the key concept of training **specificity**—target your training to your goals.

How to Apply

The principle of specificity may have begun with athletes in strength and conditioning, but we can extrapolate it to an even more precise level in your hypertrophy training. The applied scientific theory states that by targeting a variety of stresses that stimulate muscle to increase in size, your full growth potential can be realized (Haun et al. 2019).

More specifically, research suggests that there are two main types of muscular hypertrophy: **metabolic hypertrophy** and **structural hypertrophy**.* Metabolic hypertrophy is the result of adaptations induced by straining stresses that are related to short-term energy production and metabolic waste removal. Structural hypertrophy is initiated by muscle tension and damage stresses, resulting in larger and tougher muscle. By specifically targeting each component for growth, you'll achieve the greatest overall muscle development. For you, this means using different combinations of training variables discussed in key 2 to cause specific stresses and induce both metabolic and structural growth.

Hypertrophy Note

You're not just training for growth. You're using precise training techniques to target different *types* of growth.

Metabolic Growth

Muscle is a very metabolically active tissue, consisting of cells that are filled with water. Hard exercise exposes muscle cells to metabolic waste, which is a signal that the hardworking muscle isn't able to keep up with energy demand. This is analogous to an internal combustion engine. We create an explosive amount of energy to power our vehicles, but the chemical reactions produce a lot of chemical waste.

For the sake of practicality, the theory of connective tissue hypertrophy (Haun et al. 2019) is addressed via structural growth, which is a term that combines the theoretical stress stimuli of muscle tension and damage (Wackerhage et al. 2019).

Although our biochemical waste is not at all toxic, it does cause muscle to fatigue (as opposed to running out of energy). The good news is that it also serves as a stress stimulus, which causes the muscle to adapt via an increase in muscle energy stores and metabolism-related proteins. The important result is that you'll experience these adaptations as increased muscle size. Metabolic hypertrophy is also known as **sarcoplasmic hypertrophy**.

Applied Example

One great example of metabolic growth happens in response to blood flow restriction training. In this example, a tourniquet is applied to the upper portion of the limb while light resistance training is performed (Mattocks et al. 2018). The idea is to limit the amount of blood moving out of the muscle, while allowing blood flow into the muscle. Among the resulting effects, this causes a buildup of metabolic by-products from the working muscle, which serves as a great stress stimulus for the muscle to adapt.

Structural Growth

This targeted adaptation is thought to be initiated by microscopic muscle damage or tension (aka load) stress stimuli. The muscle adapts by increasing the quantity of proteins related to muscle contraction and overall structure, which you'll experience as increased size. Structural hypertrophy is also known as **myofibrillar hypertrophy** (see figure 2.5).

Although it exemplifies this type of hypertrophy, heavy eccentric training is one of the most untapped training tools in your arsenal. Consider that nearly every rep has an eccentric component during which we're stronger, but all the focus is on the effort of the concentric part. In fact, the load of the entire set is limited by this concentric strength, which is known as the **concentric**

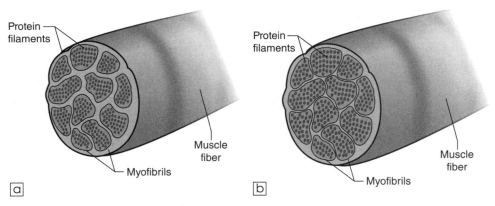

Figure 2.5   Myofibrillar hypertrophy.

constraint. As a reminder, the resistance chosen for *every set* is limited to how much force you can produce during part of the concentric phase.

Despite our higher **force potential** (aka strength) during the eccentric part of the rep, we almost always exert *less* force eccentrically. This strength gap means that we have a huge amount of force that we're leaving on the table—*every rep*. The great news is that we have a huge opportunity for hypertrophy if we can figure out how to take advantage of this. In upcoming sections you'll see how to tap into this paradox and accelerate growth.

WRAP-UP

You've likely begun this chapter with an understanding of targeted anatomy, and with the addition of three more key targets, the future of your arm development should be taking shape. The groundwork for your personalized application of training parameters (starting with frequency, intensity, time, type, volume, and progression) was described early and will continue to develop throughout subsequent chapters.

The general concept of adaptive targeting may seem complicated at first, but it should fundamentally upgrade the perception of recovery adaptation. This will be helpful for training, of course, but also for the application of recovery techniques discussed in chapter 8.

Finally, with precise microtargeting you can personalize your training and stimulate the two types of muscle growth. This is a beefy chapter, no doubt, but by applying these concepts, the same will be said of your arms.*

*I just added cheese to the menu.

Whole-Body Integration

I can hear it now: "Hey, brah, I just want swole pipes. Why bother with the rest?" As with every other component of this work, the answer is *to strategically optimize and personalize your arm training and physique development*.

Many years ago, when I started lifting, a colleague told me, "You really only need to focus on chest and biceps—it's all anyone cares about." I took this advice to heart and ended up with an imbalanced physique and more shoulder issues than I care to mention. Worst of all, those shoulder issues prevented me from training *any* muscle until I resolved the problem (from which, ironically, my biceps and pectoralis development suffered).

This old-school thinking is still applied to today's strength training. If you've ever seen images of people who have injected synthol (an oil that causes temporary localized muscle swelling) into their biceps, you know how absurd it can look to have large muscle imbalances. Similarly, albeit to a lesser degree, trying to look good by training only a few muscle groups results in an awkwardly imbalanced and horribly unflattering look. It's important to focus on building your arms without neglecting the rest of your body. The uptake here is that you'll improve the function (and look) of your entire body, which will help to facilitate your optimal arm development.

BULLET PROOFING YOUR BODY

One lesson I learned from my initial arm-focused myopia is that the body is an incredibly well-integrated machine. We can focus on muscle groups, yes, but never truly isolate. This is especially true for your goal of bulked-up limbs, and its relationship to two seemingly unrelated muscle groups—the shoulder joint and the core. These happen to be the most common sites of training-induced physical injury in the Western world. If you can keep these areas healthy, you're well on your way to quickly reaching and then surpassing your goals.

Although we can't directly claim injury prevention, the term *bullet proofing* can be used to describe how you can make these areas stronger, tougher, and more resilient. The definition of *bullet proof* says it all: *making something impervious to damage by means of prevention*. We'll bullet proof the shoulders and core by using a two-pronged approach of (1) specific exercises and (2) stabilizing tension. The bonus is that this approach also comes with a side of physique enhancement.

The shoulder is the most mobile joint in the body, but this mobility comes at the cost of stability. Imagine that the head of the humerus sitting in its socket is analogous to a golf ball sitting on a tee. This is pretty bad, but Dr. Justin Farnsworth, an expert who has seen tons of beat-down joints, believes that this doesn't go far enough. He states that a better way of describing the stability of the shoulder is "More like a ball, tenuously balanced on a dolphin's nose." (Justin Farnsworth, pers. comm.).

Practically speaking, this means that we need to be aware that this joint is particularly susceptible to injury. This is partly because of our chronic bad posture of which even I am guilty, as well as exaggerated emphasis on pressing movements (i.e., the mirror muscles—anterior muscles that we like to see in our reflection). Remember that the major arm muscles cross the shoulder joint, so you have another reason to focus on shoulder bullet proofing for optimal arm development.

The following three exercises may be challenging at first, especially if you've been neglecting your upper back work (as most of us have). As you begin to get the feel for each, work your way up to three sets each workout.

Tips

- Remember that these are intended for activation, not exhaustion.
- If you're really looking to fix a hunched posture and to bullet proof, you should consider performing these every day. This is especially for those of you who spend 12 hours a day huddled over a keyboard while working, playing video games, writing an arm training book, and so on.

SideBarr

The shoulder complex is a series of four joints, largely held together by the shoulder blade (aka [also known as] the scapula). This single bone has 17 muscle attachments! These muscles span all the way from your forearm to your lower back. This incredible level of integration helps to show that there's no such thing as isolation training—if you're focusing on one muscle, you're affecting many others in some way.

In order to help stabilize the shoulder and offset the huge volume of overhead and especially frontal pressing that everyone does, we'll draw heavily from the insights explored through the Pain Free Performance Specialist Certification (PPSC). After nearly 30 years of lifting, lessons from the PPSC have had the biggest overall impact on my training, and they rank number 1 on my list of things I wish I had known sooner. The first of these comes from PPSC founder Dr. John Rusin and is aptly named the Rusin three-way banded shoulder saver. It's simple, but it is also a life-altering component of **preworkout activation**.

Banded Over and Back

Setup

1. Grab a light band with an overhand grip and your elbows extended.
2. The elbows will naturally flex as needed throughout this shoulder and upper back-focused movement.

Execution

1. Raise your hands back and over your head while moving the arms into external rotation (*a*).
2. Once overhead, drop your hands down behind you as you retract your shoulder blades (i.e., pull them together) (*b*).
3. Reverse the direction to return to the starting position.

Coaching Tip

Use a light band and focus on the quality of the movement.

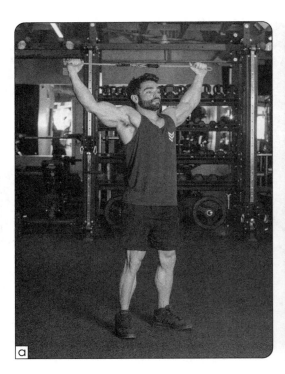
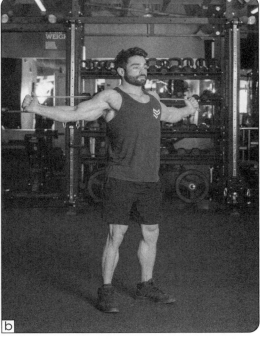

Banded Face Pull

Setup

1. Anchor the band at chin height.
2. Grab the other end of the band with the fingers of both of your hands.
3. Facing the anchor, step back to establish tension with your arms straight out in front of you. Your forearms should be roughly parallel with each other and the ground (*a*).

Execution

1. Drive your elbows back and externally rotate the humerus so that your forearms approach vertical to the ground (*b*).
2. End the concentric portion when your hands are beside your face, between your forehead and chin..
3. Reverse the movement for the eccentric portion.

Coaching Tip

Keep a light but secure grip on the band to ensure that your arms do not become excessively involved.

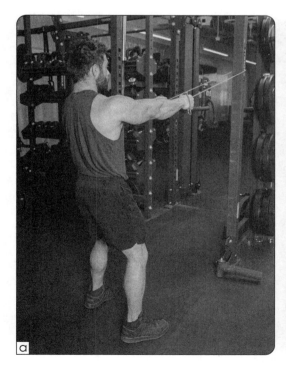

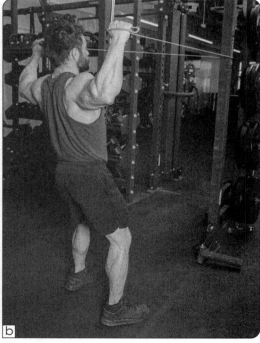

Banded Pull-Apart

Setup

1. Put your head through the center of a band so it hangs like a chain around your neck.
2. Grab the far end with both hands using an overhand grip, so that your forearms are roughly parallel to each other.
3. Extend your elbows and bring your arms up to shoulder height in front of you (*a*).
4. Make sure your palms are facing the ground.

Execution

1. Abduct your arms to pull the band apart, by squeezing your back musculature.
2. As you're abducting, rotate the wrists so that your thumbs are pointing up by the end of the concentric portion (*b*).
3. Reverse the movements for the eccentric portion.

Coaching Tip

It's surprisingly common to lose core tension when performing this standing exercise. Be aware of this and maintain stabilizing tension throughout.

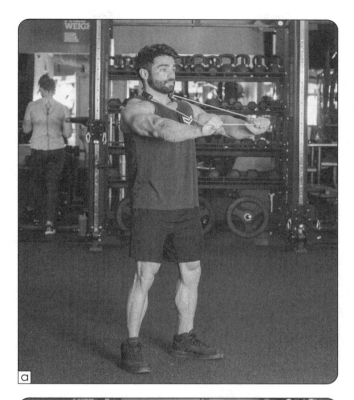

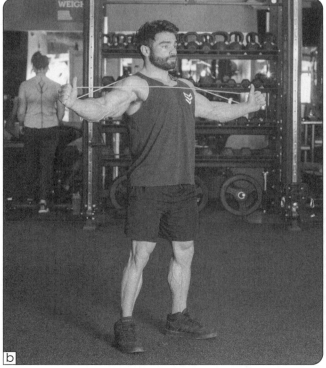

CORE PREPARATION EXERCISES

In spite of my haunting hours with cadavers in the anatomy lab, it never fails to amaze me how integrated our entire muscular system is. One of the best examples is your core, which is involved in nearly every movement you do. This is essential to not only understand but also to come to *appreciate* when you're targeting arm training.

I've known a few otherwise healthy people who have injured their lower backs by heaving up that last rep during a set of barbell biceps curls. If you're thinking, "That's stupid; it would never happen to me," know that each individual thought the exact same thing, right up until it happened.

One common reason for this type of injury (and many others) is a general lack of core strength. We can be confident about this sweeping claim by identifying that the core musculature ranges from front to back and side to side, from nipples to knees. Using this broad definition helps to reinforce the idea that our muscles and their connections are a complex, integrated network. As we come to truly appreciate this concept, we'll be able to take full advantage for optimal muscular development.

Developing core strength will help you to perform heavier arm exercises, *and pretty much everything else you do in life*.

As part of preworkout activation, you'll come to dominate two powerful exercises: modified bird dogs and dead bugs.

Tips

- These movements are most helpful when you continually try to improve your form, each rep. Start the exercise by moving one limb at a time and try to improve the technique with each. When you develop single limb movement mastery, you can perform with two limbs. Although it is common for people to jump the gun and start with the two-limb version, it is important to earn this progression. In doing so, your execution of the movement with simultaneous opposite limbs will be much higher quality and subsequently far more effective, which will feel like a major accomplishment.

- If you're new to these exercises, keep in mind that quality is king. It doesn't matter if you're performing only three reps at a time, as long as you're getting better with each rep. You can personalize your execution of these movements by using the key performance indicator of movement quality, rather than a predetermined number of reps. Once movement quality fails to improve on two consecutive reps, it's likely that fatigue has set in, and it's time to call an end to the set.

Bird Dog (Modified)

Setup

1. Start on your hands and knees (aka quadruped position).
2. Screw your hands into the ground by firmly planting them and then trying to rotate them outward. A similar technique is used for many lower body exercises and is described in Put the Screw On (see page 48).
3. Establish stabilizing tension in your hips and core.

Execution—Arm

1. Bring one arm up to 90 degrees at the shoulder and elbow.
2. Make a fist with your palm facing the midline of your body (i.e., the neutral position) (*a*).
3. Punch forward by flexing the shoulder and extending the elbow. Simultaneously rotate the wrist so that the palm of the fist is facing the ground (i.e., pronate it).
4. In the end position, make sure your biceps muscle is beside your ear.
5. Reverse the direction for the eccentric portion.

Execution—Leg

1. Extend your hip and try to maintain a horizontal shin angle throughout.
2. Very lightly drag your big toe along the ground as you drive back and raise it only an inch to complete the concentric portion of the exercise (*b*).
3. Reverse the movement for the eccentric portion.

Coaching Tips

- This is not an arm or leg exercise; it is a stability-and-control-while-moving exercise.
- Only move the limb you're intentionally trying to move. Everything else should be rock solid.
- The amount of tension you want to generate can be shown with the following cue: you should be trying to grip the ground so hard that if someone were to turn it upside down, you'd be able to cling to it.
- For simultaneous limb work, try to create the greatest distance between your hand and your big toe. That will prevent you from creating the excessive lower back curve that you see on Instagram. This is the time for movement quality, not for gaining followers!

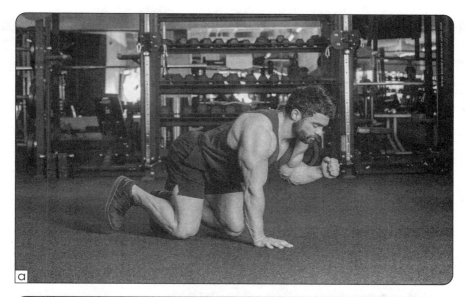

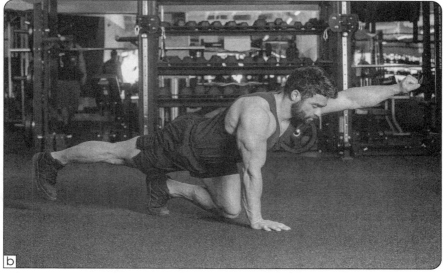

Dead Bug

Setup

1. Lie on your back with your thighs and arms vertical
2. Bend your knees at 90 degrees and extend your elbows (*a*).

Execution—Arm

1. Extend one shoulder so that it ends near the top of your head as your hand touches the ground.
2. Reverse the direction for the concentric portion.

Execution—Leg

1. Extend at one hip while keeping your shin parallel to the ground so that your knee naturally extends (*b*).
2. When your heel taps the ground, reverse the direction for the concentric portion.

Coaching Tips

- This is not an arm or leg exercise; it is a stability-and-control-while-moving exercise.
- Only move the limb you're intentionally trying to move. Everything else should be rock solid.
- Your torso is fully supported by the ground, which makes this the perfect time to focus on bracing and breathing while moving your limbs.

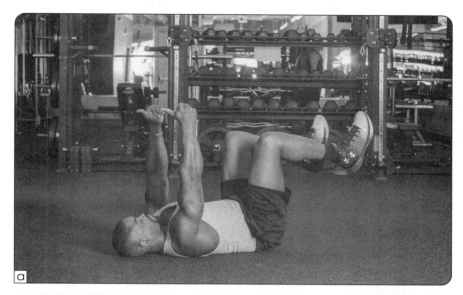

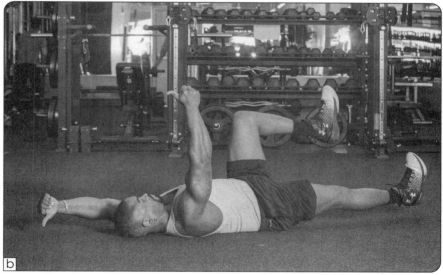

KEY 5: TARGETED FOCUS

The concept of bullet proofing dovetails nicely with the fifth and final key target (the first four keys were discussed in chapters 1 and 2). It begins by activating your most neglected training tool: your brain. Rather than mindlessly moving iron (which we usually do), you can use your attentional focus to significantly upgrade your training stimulus. Once you experience this and the subsequent results, you'll never go back to traditional meathead (i.e., all muscle, no brain) workouts.

This key target is so big it comes in two phases. Phase I is all about creating internal tension to stabilize your body and allow it to perform optimally. Phase II challenges your instincts to get the most out of each muscle contraction.

As a reminder of each of the five key targets, which were discussed in this chapter and chapters 1 and 2, they have been compiled and are summarized here:

1. *Anatomically targeted training.* Understanding your physical anatomy and that of resistance training, so you can then optimize

2. *Targeted training parameters.* The various ways through which the training stimulus can be manipulated

3. *Adaptive targeting.* Stress stimulus, stress response, recovery, and adaptation (aka four-phase gains)

4. *Precision microtargeting.* Training to stimulate both metabolic growth and structural growth for maximal muscle development

5. *Targeted focus.* Whole-body stability (phase I) and internal locus of focus (phase II)

Focus Phase I: Stabilizing Tension

This phase is all about creating stability for your entire body, which might help to mitigate injury risk, but can also make your lifts better. The central idea is that your body has internal sensors that detect how stable you are in a particular position, which then affects your strength. For example, imagine standing on an unstable surface like a pair of inflatable discs. How much force could you put into an overhead barbell press in this state? Now swap the discs for a solid rubber floor and imagine the same scenario. You can almost *feel* the greater strength and stability with the latter.

This change in your ability to produce force is internally regulated by your nervous system. It's a protective mechanism to ensure that you're not exerting too much force in an unstable and potentially injurious position. Why would your body subject itself to risky movements if you're about as safe as Bambi on ice? The body likes to feel stable—that's when it allows you to perform maximally. We can use this knowledge to enhance performance with each and every set. If we increase this level of stability on every lift, we'll be able to generate greater force and have better overall performance, which translates into muscular development. Remember: *be stable, be strong.*

Put the Screw On

One way to create stabilizing tension throughout your body is by "screwing" your feet into the ground when standing. This happens by trying to turn your feet out (externally rotating, creating torque) while they are firmly planted. Squeeze your gluteus and inner thigh muscles (i.e., your adductors) for maximal effect. This base of support establishes the foundation for maximal strength.

Apply this technique to lower body exercises by thinking of the eccentric portion of the movement as a controlled pulling down (during a squat, for example), as opposed to passively dropping down. It may feel a bit unusual at first, but you'll soon come to love the stability, the control, and the gains.

Brace Yourself

The next step is probably going to change your life. It's called **bracing** and was popularized by one of my earliest mentors in strength and conditioning, Dr. Stu McGill, who also happens to be a world's expert in lower back and core function.

Traditional bracing has been described as taking a deep breath and holding it, in an attempt to establish tension throughout your core. An updated, and more accurate description is to take a breath in and pretend that you're about the be punched in the stomach. You can do this right now and *feel* it. That resulting tension can be applied during a lift to help to stabilize your core and ultimately the rest of your body.

The amount of bracing tension can be regulated based on how much stability you need during a given exercise. If you're performing a maximal-effort back squat, you want to hold near-maximal tension. Contrast this with a set of seated calf raises, for which you can let out more breath to scale down the tension. Note that you're not holding your breath the entire time. You might briefly hold it during the heaviest portion of the concentric phase, but the goal is to maintain a braced core while breathing as needed.

Tip

If you're a chest breather (i.e., your chest inflates rather than your abdomen), you will have an additional challenge of learning to use your diaphragm to draw breath (aka belly breathing). That's because bracing pulls your rib cage down for stability, so the diaphragm is forced (or allowed) to do all the work of breathing. It's beyond the scope of this book to go into significant detail, but your entire body will benefit from learning to breathe through your diaphragm. You'll find a strategy to take advantage of this powerful physiology in chapter 8, Recovery Optimization.

Shoulder Stability

The final part of stabilizing tension, which is especially important for arm training, is stabilizing the shoulder by isometrically contracting your pectoralis and latissimus dorsi muscles during the set. When you're doing isolation work, the new level of stability provided through this squeeze will immediately be a game changer for your arms. The first couple of times you try this it may seem impossible to imagine a scenario when this will become automatic. In my experience with clients and athletes, this is one of the fastest adaptations our mind and body pick up. There's something very telling about that. Stated simply: it might feel unnatural at first, but our body really likes it and is quick to adopt it.

Summary of Phase I Focus—Internal Stability

1. Screwing into the ground
2. Bracing
3. Shoulders (pectoralis and latissimus dorsi muscles)

It's important to remember that you're doing this to provide immediate performance enhancement, as well as training longevity. It may take you a few weeks to really feel comfortable with stabilizing tension, but performing this with every set gives you a ton of practice and the results come fast. It's so effective that you shouldn't be surprised to find yourself bracing during everyday activities (e.g., picking up bags, dogs, cars, etc.). In fact, achieving this level of automatic activation allows you to progress to focus phase II. This quote from Dr. John Rusin concisely explains the need for developing internal tension: "Your goal is to make light weight feel heavy, so you can make heavy weight feel light." (John Rusin, pers. comm.). Stated differently, if you make the effort to develop stability today, you'll be much stronger tomorrow.

Focus Phase II: Mind–Muscle Connection

The scientific term for phase II focus is **locus of focus** and refers to where you place your attention during each rep. Think about your most recent lift and try to recall. Was your attention focused on squeezing the muscle, which ultimately moves the load, or were you laser locked on moving the resistance itself (e.g., a dumbbell)? The universal answer is the latter, which provides another exciting opportunity for arm growth.

We have limited capacity for attention, so it's important that you first master focus phase I before progressing. Once you're able to create tension and stability throughout your body almost automatically, you're ready to take full advantage of this next level of focus. Research has shown that for maximal hypertrophy, you should *put your attention into squeezing the muscle to move the load* throughout the entire rep (Schoenfeld et al. 2018).

It might sound obvious, but it's actually counterintuitive. Our instinct is to make things easier by focusing on moving the load. How many times have you found yourself fighting to just get the bar up on your last rep? Sure, it may feel hard at that point, but what about every other rep until then? Did those preceding reps contribute to growth stimulation, or were they simply filler so you could stimulate at the end of the set?

Intentionally contracting the muscle is known as an ***internal* locus of focus**, because you're focused on your active muscles rather than an external implement. It's great for hypertrophy because it makes our muscle contraction *less* efficient, which is exactly what we want. This inefficiency creates greater metabolic waste during the set, which is a stress stimulus we explored in chapter 2. This translates into faster fatigue during the set, so you may have to drop the weight a little at first. Uh-oh. Using a lighter load sounds horrible, doesn't it? But recall from the key of precision microtargeting that your training objective is to induce optimal stress stimulus on the muscle. In this case, the powerfully focused stress stimulus targets metabolic growth.

So, if you're training for muscle development, ignore the "devil" of your short-term ego and stick to what you'll soon see working. If you're still wary, remind your ego that a recent analysis of hypertrophy research showed that high- and low-load resistance are equally effective for gains (Schoenfeld et al. 2017)—and that's even *without* the focus-based boost that you'll soon be using.

Don't worry; your strength will come. For strength training phases, you'll employ an ***external* locus of focus**, which is all about moving the load itself. Note that this is what most people do most of the time, *if* they're even focused on the training at hand (which they're often not).

STOP WARMING UP

One of the best kept training secrets lies in executing a dramatic paradigm shift for what is traditionally thought of as a warm-up. The reality is that when done right, it's probably the best performance booster we have at our disposal.

Somewhere along the way our warm-up became little more than an obligation. It morphed into "that thing we do because someone told us it might help prevent injuries." This is a wasted opportunity, every workout.

No more.

In order to take full advantage, you will come to think of the warm-up as the preparation phase, or activation phase of your workout. Rather than simply getting your body warm and preventing something that will probably never happen to you anyway (i.e., injuries), your focused activation phase will help you perform better, both mentally and physically. *This* is the time to get your head in the game, not chat about Instagram posts or how much alcohol you drank last night.

You will still want to perform traditional physical preparation, like brief cardiovascular exercise to help get your blood moving, and dynamic stretching, etc. But after that, you're going to treat your activation as though you're getting ready for a fight. No more lazy stretching while you lie around talking about your weekend. This idea was best summed up by PPSC Chief Content Officer David Otey, "If you want to perform optimally, you need to prepare optimally." (David Otey, pers. comm.).

You will execute your bullet proofing movements with intent and focus on quality. You will practice the exercises that you are going to perform on that day, before you have anything more than body-weight resistance. These activation exercises are not meant to replace exercise-specific warm-up sets of increasing load (e.g., a set of curls with 45 pounds [20.4 kg], then another with 65 pounds [29.5 kg], before moving on to your work set), but the body-weight movement will come to enhance those loaded sets.

Performing without load allows you to focus on creating internal tension (focus phase I) and prepares you to execute the loaded movement with maximal force or speed, without the nagging fear of injury. This is where you'll develop even more confidence to perform that day. You will establish the mind–muscle connection that gives you the mental and physical confidence to crush each lift. If performed with intent and focus, you will feel the difference, immediately.

Your warm-up is dead. Long live activation!

Example of a Squat-Focused Preworkout Activation Plan

- Five minutes on the treadmill
- Three-way Rusin shoulder saver
- Modified bird dogs
- Dead bugs
- Focused body-weight squats
- Jumping jacks

STRATEGIC WHOLE-BODY TRAINING: MOVEMENTS AND EXERCISES

We need to establish some ground rules about optimal lifting. For example, if the central tenet of this book is to optimize your arm musculature, then any indirect training components must *at least* not interfere with this. That's only fair, right? But if we're more strategic about the process, a more advanced goal would be to choose exercises that actually enhance both short- and long-term arm development. We're getting warmer.

The best-case scenario would be if this training also enhanced long-term strength, as well as arm and overall physique development, while also mitigating risk of injury. If you're still reading, it's likely because you've guessed that we're going with the final option: ultimate arm training.

Body Part–Specific Exercises

As a final note regarding your personalized physique training, it's possible that you may want to add more traditional body part–specific exercises, like calf raises or shrugs. Before you throw them in blindly, it's important to first see how your body responds to the program without them. Considering that many of these strategic exercises may be new, and you're developing your ability to brace and focus on contracting muscles, you may be surprised by their whole-body impact.

This was best exemplified by a client who was desperate to grow his calves, while integrating this whole-body program. In spite of the warnings, he threw heavy calf raises into the program along with a variety of novel lower body work. The result? His calves were so sore that limping to the toilet became the extent of his physical ability for the next three days. For this reason, we'll focus on arm exercises, as well as strategically chosen movement-based exercises that will facilitate arm development, discussed in the following sections.

SIX FOUNDATIONAL MOVEMENTS

The exercise selection is strategically developed to boost your arm-centric program, while still hitting the *six* **foundational human movement patterns**: *squat, hinge, lunge, push, pull, and carry*. To better appreciate their importance, we'll identify the selected exercises and the rationale for their inclusion before adding them into programs (in later chapters).

Foundational Movement 1: Squat

Although we have an exercise generally called a squat (typically referring to barbell back squat), it's more accurate to think of it as a movement with many variations. This is more of a knee-dominant movement that often results in the shins and torso being nearly parallel at the end of the range of motion (ROM).

Goblet Squat

This pure squat movement allows you to focus on creating internal tension and controlling every aspect of the exercise.

Equipment

Kettlebell or dumbbell

Setup

1. Grab one horn of the kettlebell (KB) with each hand using a neutral (palms-facing) grip.
2. Stand in a comfortable squat stance and bring the hands up to chest height.
3. Squeeze the pectoralis and latissimus dorsi muscles to create tension (*a*).

Execution

1. Draw your body down by flexing at the knees, ankles, and hips.
2. Stop when reaching your squat depth, such as the tops of your thighs parallel to the ground (*b*).
3. Reverse the direction for the concentric movement.

Coaching Tips

- Keep the shoulders tight and the implement locked against your upper chest. You'll be able to tell whether you're providing enough stabilizing tension (by cocontracting your latissimus dorsi and pectoralis muscles), because you should end up with a bit of an upper body pump by the time you complete the set.
- Perform in front of a mirror to gain visual cues about your technique and depth.

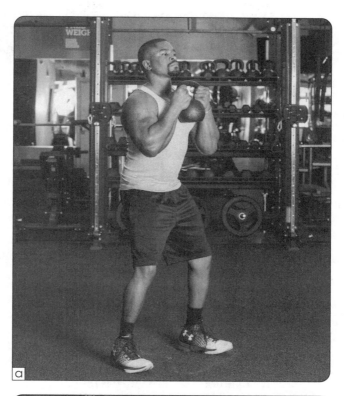

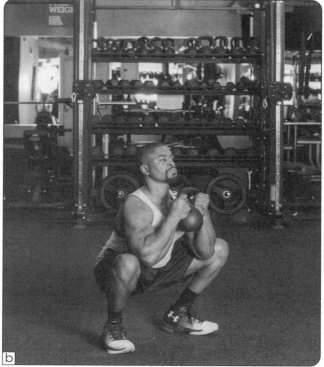

Elevated Narrow-Stance, Quad-Focused, Single-Rack Squat

Equipment

Kettlebell (alternative: light barbell) and two weight plates

Setup

1. Grab the handle of the KB so the bell hangs down, resting against the back (aka posterior) of your forearm.
2. The "rack" position consists of having your arm nearly vertical and pressed firmly into your side. The elbow will be flexed nearly maximally, so that the forearm is also nearly vertical.
3. Your hand with the KB should be just in front of your pectoralis muscles.
4. Using a narrow stance and feet pointed forward (parallel to each other), elevate your heels on plates to place more of the load on the anterior foot and toes (*a*).

Execution

1. Draw your body down by flexing at the knees, ankles, and hips.
2. Stop the eccentric movement when you reach a deep squat, as long as you remain pain-free (*b*).
3. Reverse the direction for the concentric movement.
4. Extend your nonworking arm; you can place it at your side, slightly abducted. This will be an organic arm position to help with balance and should not be overcoached.

Coaching Tips

- This is a specific hypertrophy-based exercise that targets the teardrop muscle (aka vastus medialis) like no other.
- Although front loading is ideal to maintain more of a pure squat movement, grip or shoulder fatigue might require you to use a light barbell on your back.

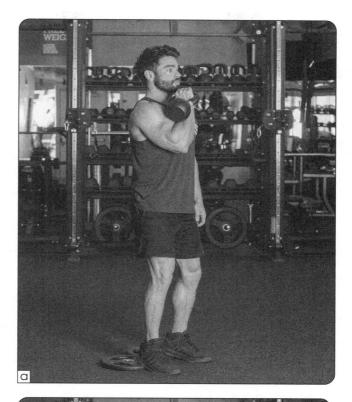

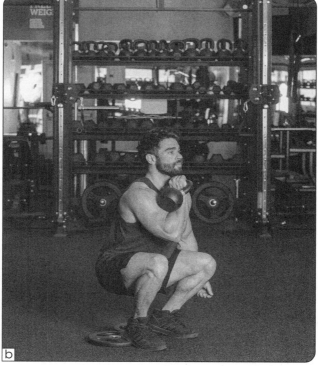

Foundational Movement 2: Hinge

The hinge is often described simply as bending over, which conjures images of imminent back pain. A more accurate description is pushing your hips back to bend at the waist. Even this subtle shift in focus from lower back to hips causes a huge change in how this movement is perceived and performed.

Figure 3.1 exemplifies the differences between the squat and hinge movement patterns, along with representative exercises that fit along the spectrum. This also helps to illustrate why, although barbell back squats and deadlifts have their places, we are focused on purer versions of these movements (i.e., goblet squats and Romanian deadlifts [RDLs]) as part of our focus on arm training.

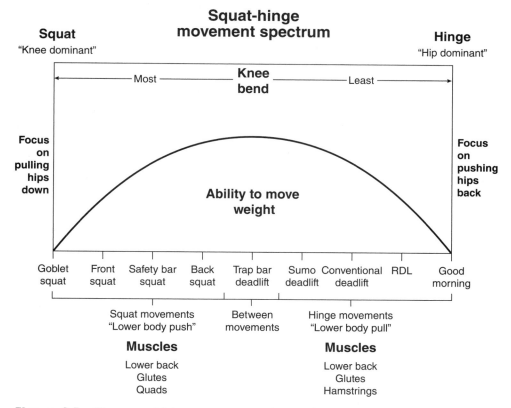

Figure 3.1 The squat-hinge movement spectrum.

Reprinted by permission from Dr. John Rusin.

Romanian Deadlift

The RDL is a pure hinge movement that allows you to focus on whole-body stability and really squeeze the entire posterior chain (i.e., muscles running from the back of your head all the way down to your heels).

Equipment

Barbell (alternative: anything)

Setup

1. Grab the barbell at slightly wider than shoulder width with an overhand grip.
2. Flex your knees slightly and maintain this flexion throughout (*a*).

Execution

1. Squeeze your glutes and hamstrings to push your hips back to hinge.
2. Allow the load to hang close to your thighs, knees, and shins throughout (*b*).
3. Stop the movement at a comfortable depth, such as when the bar reaches the bottom of your kneecap.
4. Reverse the movement to perform the concentric portion.

Coaching Tips

- Although maintaining a flat back or slight lordotic curve is common to nearly every exercise, it is worth emphasizing here.
- Under normal circumstances, your grip strength won't limit your RDL load, but it may be an issue because of your arm and grip-specific training. Use wrist straps or a hook grip to get around this at first. Your strength should increase quickly enough that it won't be a problem for long.

Note

A hook grip is commonly used by Olympic weightlifters to move heavy loads very quickly, but in a pinch, it can be used for any grip-limiting exercise. It consists of first wrapping your palm and thumb tightly around the implement (e.g., a barbell) and then closing this grip by wrapping your fingers *over* your thumb. You then use your fingers to further squeeze your thumb into the bar. It doesn't feel great on your thumb, but it's effective and you get used to it. Figure 3.2 illustrates the most common types of bar grips.

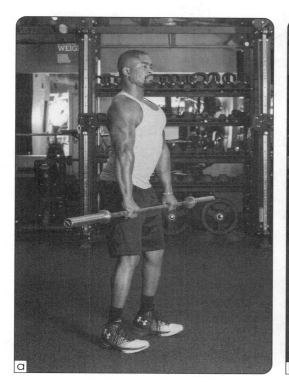
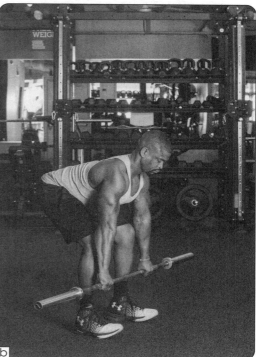

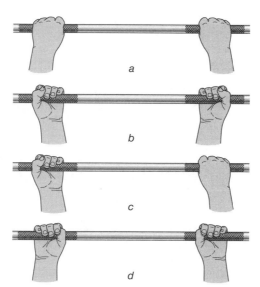

Figure 3.2 Types of bar grips: (*a*) pronated, (*b*) supinated, (*c*) alternated, and (*d*) hook (posterior view).

Reprinted by permission from NSCA, "Exercise Technique for Free Weight and Machine Training," by S. Caufield and D. Berninger, in *Essentials of Strength Training and Conditioning,* 4th ed. (Champaign, IL: Human Kinetics, 2016), 352.

Ball Hamstring Curl and Hip Extension

You may recall that our arm muscles cross two joints (elbow and shoulder). Our leg muscles are anatomically similar. To address this idea, just as we do with arms, this exercise gives us a twofer—it hits the hamstring muscles across two joints for the price of one.

Equipment

Stability ball (aka Swiss ball)

Setup

1. Lie face up with your heels and ankles on the ball.
2. Start with your pelvis on the ground (*a*).

Execution

1. Progressively extend your hips and flex your knees to drive your pelvis upward. This will roll the ball underneath you (*b*).
2. When you can no longer move concentrically, reverse the direction for the eccentric portion.

Coaching Tips

- Perform the movements at each joint simultaneously (e.g., curl the ball and extend your hips at the same time).
- You will likely need to reset the starting position a couple of times during the set, because each rep could push the ball farther away from you.

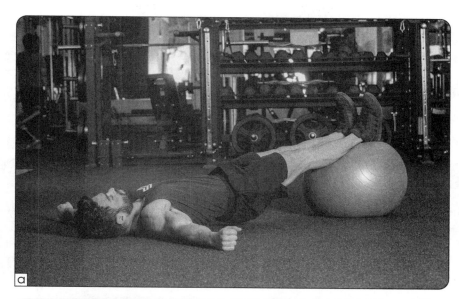

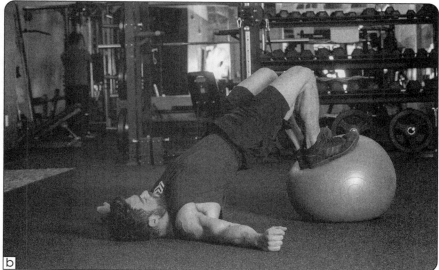

Foundational Movement 3: Lunge

Although potentially confusing, it is easiest to describe a lunge broadly as single leg–focused work that can fall into one of the following two primary movements (both fall into the movement category of lunge):

1. Lunging, involves lifting and moving a foot during the exercise
2. Split squats, in which the feet do not move

Reverse Lunge

This exercise is often easier on the knees than forward lunging, during which people (like me) often place too much emphasis on the rear leg (and after many years grind their anterior cruciate ligament into a fine powder). Rear lunging provides all of the benefits with less potential for pain.

Equipment

Body weight (alternative: dumbbells)

Setup

1. Establish your bottom position so you know roughly how far you are stepping back during the exercise. Your working hip, knee, and ankle joints will be at roughly 90 degrees each (aka 3-90). Note the placement and position of the rear foot and leg.
2. Stand with your feet slightly wider than shoulder-width apart (*a*).

Execution

1. Step backward as you draw yourself down using the tension of the working leg (*b*).
2. Contract the musculature of the working leg and hip to bring yourself back to standing.

Coaching Tips

- Your rear leg should only serve as a kickstand for support.
- Ensure that you're using your working leg for the concentric movement— ignore the temptation to push off with your rear leg.

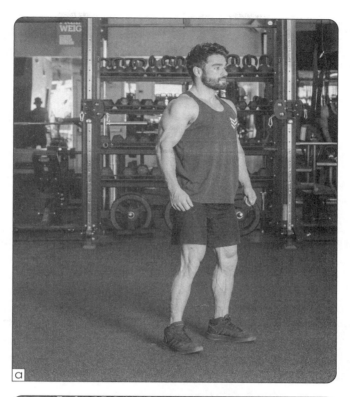

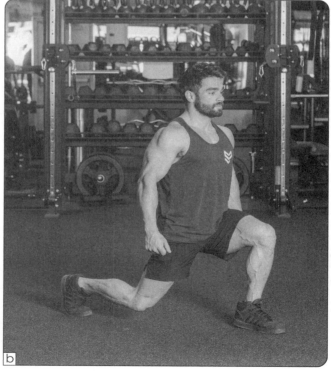

Bulgarian Split Squat

Once you have the technique mastered, you can really load this exercise up for a powerful growth stimulus.

Equipment

Dumbbells (alternative: body weight or kettlebells)

Setup

1. Establish your foot position by first finding your bottom position.
2. With the support leg behind you elevated on a bench, your working leg will be at roughly 3-90.

Execution

1. Starting with your knee fully extended (*a*), draw yourself down using the musculature of your working leg.
2. When you reach your established ending position (*b*), use your working limb (including hip) to perform the concentric portion.
3. Allow your arms to hang straight down at your sides throughout.

Coaching Tips

- Your rear leg should only serve as a kickstand for support.
- Ensure that you're using your working leg for the concentric portion of the exercise—ignore the temptation to push off with your rear leg.
- The top of your rear foot can be used for additional support if balance or toe pain are problematic. Just be sure to use a padded bench, folded towel, etc. under that very bony part of your foot.

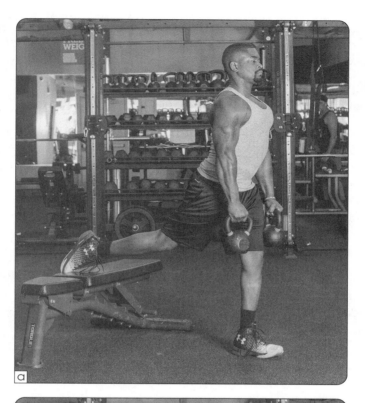

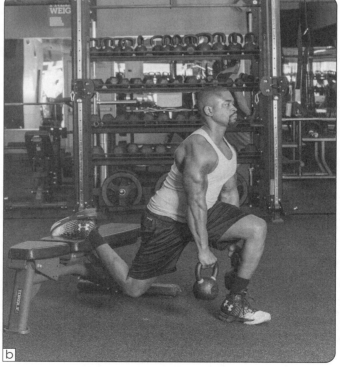

Foundational Movement 4: Push

The upper body push is broken down into the following two movement planes:

1. Horizontal, which can be represented by the bench press
2. Vertical, is exemplified by an overhead press

Pressing is going to create the greatest challenge to the arm-training program because you're already doing so much of it during arm sessions. This is a great example of the need for strategic exercise selection and integration.

The dumbbell pectoralis fly exhibits a near-perfect opposite-strength curve from the dumbbell lateral raise discussed in chapter 1. They both have an extreme force delta, but the fly provides the greatest load at the start of the concentric portion. This is problematic for two reasons:

1. The working muscles are typically stretched at this point.
2. The shoulder joint is in a somewhat vulnerable position—especially as your arm drops below horizontal (toward the ground). Remember, your shoulder is as stable as a ball balanced on a dolphin's nose.

You might like the feel of the loaded stretch at the bottom of a fly, or you may have even been instructed to make this stretch happen, but this type of unstable loaded stretching is contraindicated.

Another problem with having this vulnerable position at the end of the eccentric ROM, which is the momentum that is commonly generated during the descent. It may happen because we're in a hurry to feel tension on the muscle, and the first half of the descent is relatively tension free. The result is that we pick up a little more speed at first and try to slow this down as we begin to feel the pectoralis and shoulder muscles working. It can be subtle, but any additional load at a vulnerable and unstable position could push us past the integrity of the joint. This can be especially true as our stabilizer muscles fatigue, when even a momentary loss in stability could result in injury in this position.

I've attempted to fix the extreme force delta and generate tension at the top of the fly, by squeezing the dumbbells together for an isometric contraction. After playing with this for a couple of years, I came to realize that we can perform an identical contraction at *any time* by simply pushing our hands together; using dumbbells does not confer a magic benefit to this action. In other words, this little trick didn't solve any the fundamental problems with the pectoralis fly.

For these reasons, performing the pectoralis fly movement with cables, elastic resistance, or machines is preferred to dumbbells. Preview: We'll explore the biggest upgrade to dumbbell flys in chapter 7 (Nontraditional Exercises).

Horizontal—Cable Fly

There's really no way to eliminate shoulder and triceps work from pressing, so the compromise will be to use banded, cable, or machine-based flys.

Equipment

Cable apparatus and D-handles (alternative: band, machine)

Setup

1. Center yourself between two opposing cable machines.
2. Set the position of the D-handles at roughly shoulder height.
3. With a hand gripping each handle, step forward as necessary so that there is tension on the pectoralis muscles in this lengthened position. Your elbows should be slightly flexed throughout to eliminate inadvertent loaded stretching of your biceps (*a*).

Execution

1. Squeeze your pectoralis muscles to bring your arms across your body in front of you (i.e., horizontally adduct your arms) (*b*).
2. Stop when you are limited by the equipment, your body, or just before you lose tension on the muscle.
3. Reverse the movement for the eccentric portion.

Coaching Tips

- As your hands approach each other, raise one and lower the other so they can pass each other, and you'll achieve a greater range of motion.
- Alternate the path of each hand (above or below) with each rep.
- Although your pectoralis muscles will be in a lengthened position at the end of the eccentric portion, avoid the temptation to stretch under load.

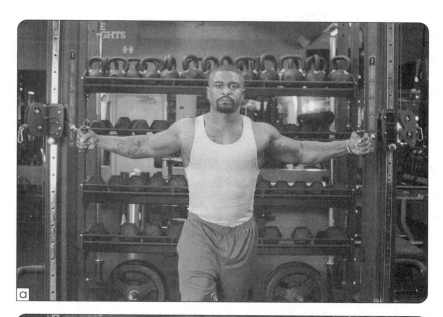

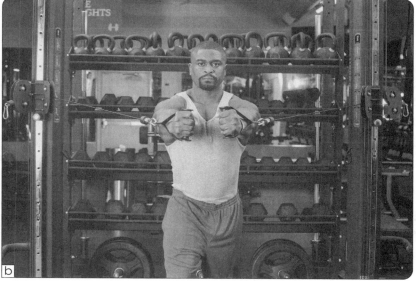

Vertical—Kettlebell Half Kneeling Bottom's-Up Press

As with horizontal pressing, the same challenge of prospective arm fatigue applies for vertical movements. For this reason, we will use the bottom's-up KB press. The bonus is that it's *not* a compromise—this exercise is one of the more effective ways to develop bulletproof shoulders.

Equipment

Kettlebell (alternative: band, dumbbell)

Setup

1. Start in a kneeling position with each knee at 90 degrees. Your front leg will be at 3-90 (i.e., 90 degrees each at the hip, knee, and ankle). Your rear leg will have the support of your knee and toes on the ground.

2. For this exercise you'll use a standard overhand grip on the handle of the KB. The difference is that the bell of the KB will remain above your hand, rather than hanging down as normal. Trying to keep the KB inverted will force you to maintain a vertical forearm and wrist (directly under the KB) throughout.

3. Your nonworking arm will have the elbow extended and can be placed at your side, slightly abducted. This will be an organic arm position to help with balance and should not be overcoached.

4. The working arm will be on the side of the rear leg.

5. The starting position and degree of elbow flexion of the working arm will be established organically by your need to keep your forearm vertical (*a*).

Execution

1. Press the KB overhead to full elbow extension (*b*).

2. Reverse the direction for the eccentric portion.

3. Keep your shoulders aligned with (directly over) your hips throughout. This will ensure that there is no unwanted rotation of the torso.

Coaching Tips

- Perform this exercise in front of a mirror for visual feedback.
- You can add variety by performing this movement with the working arm on the same side as the forward leg.
- The goal is to perform this exercise with stability and control to develop movement mastery rather than trying to push big weight. If you're used to other pressing movements, the instability of the inverted bell will make your grip the greatest challenge at first. Although you're going to feel it in your grip, this weakness might actually reflect general shoulder instability, which should improve within a training session or two. If it doesn't, you're probably going way too heavy on this move. Lastly, do not use a hook grip for this exercise. Instead, lighten the load and focus on movement mastery.

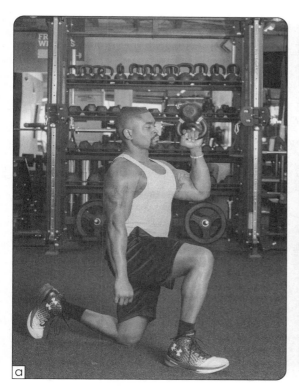 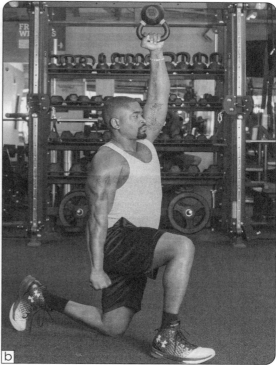

Foundational Movement 5: Pull

In direct opposition to the pressing movement is the often-neglected upper body pull. Here we're working to correct (or prevent) the traditional imbalance in pressing to pulling training volume, because let's face it, we're all too focused on the mirror muscles.

In contrast to a few torso muscles that press, we have numerous back muscles that will require a slightly higher volume to hit. This is why we'll use two horizontal pulling exercises and one for vertical.

Horizontal 1—Suspension High-Elbow Row

Equipment

Suspension trainer (alternative: barbell anchored in a squat rack)

Setup

1. If you're new to this movement, begin by setting the handles at roughly shoulder height. This can be lowered to increase resistance.
2. Establish your foot position relative to your hands, based on desired resistance. The farther forward your feet are, the more horizontal your body will be and the greater the challenge.
3. Grab the handles with an overhand (pronated) grip.
4. Start at the bottom of the movement so you can establish whole-body tension with your elbows extended and shoulders slightly flexed (*a*).

Execution

1. Drive your elbows back to perform the row, so that you end the movement with your arms roughly perpendicular to your torso (hence the descriptor, high elbow) (*b*).
2. Reverse the movement for the eccentric portion.

Coaching Tip

Work to maintain a tall spine throughout the movement; this means no cheating with the head and neck.

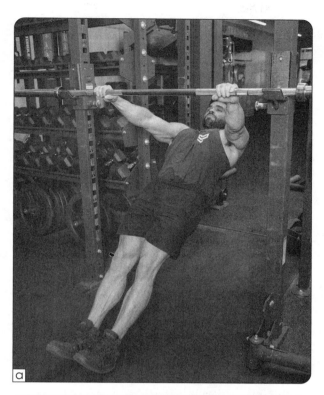

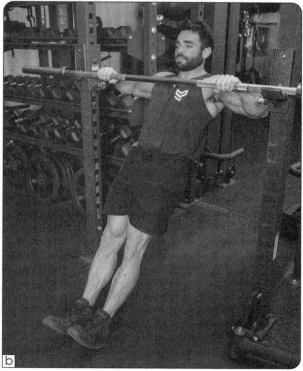

Horizontal 2—Single-Arm Seated Cable Row

This exercise is selected over a one-arm dumbbell row in order to give your core and lower body a bit of a break while allowing you to focus contracting your back musculature

Equipment

Cable apparatus and D-handle, preferably seated cable row apparatus (alternative: machine)

Setup

1. Leg position varies across machines, but the key is that you want some knee flexion, which will result in your hip being flexed at greater than 90 degrees.
2. Grab the D-handle in an overhand grip to develop tension with your shoulder flexed and elbow extended. This is the starting position (*a*).

Execution

1. Simultaneously drive your elbow back and rotate your wrist. At the end of the concentric ROM, your wrist position is in a neutral grip, so that if you were performing this with both arms, your palms would be facing each other (*b*).
2. Reverse these movements for the eccentric portion.
3. Maintain square shoulders (i.e., facing the weight stack) throughout. This means that there should be no unwanted rotation of the torso.

Coaching Tips

- Some movement of the hip is likely necessary for a full ROM at the shoulder, but resist the overwhelming urge to use hip extension to move the load.
- Although your back musculature will be in a lengthened position at the end of the eccentric movement, do not stretch the muscle under load.
- Remember that you are trying to stimulate your muscle, so the previous tips can be summarized as, watch what everybody else does and then do the opposite.

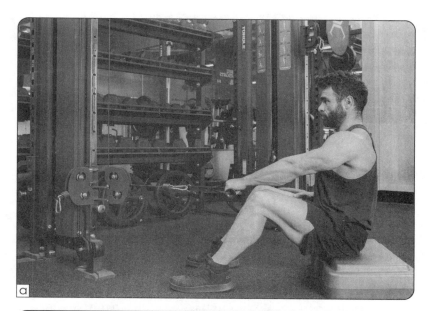

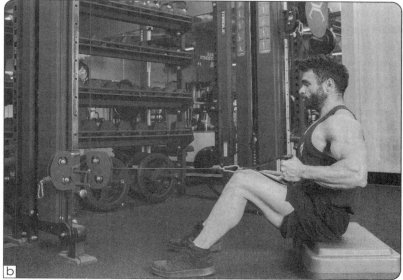

Vertical—Pull-Down, Pull-Up

This exercise can hit your back musculature differently based on the angle of your torso relative to the direction of the vertical cable. This version will use a vertical torso with the vertical cable.

Equipment

Pull-down machine

Setup

1. Establish your grip width based on where your hands will be at the end of the concentric ROM, with the goal of achieving the strongest contractions possible. As a memory aid, your forearms will be roughly vertical in this position.
2. With your arms overhead and your palms facing forward, grab the bar with your fingers (a).
3. Sit with your lower body at 3-90, and your thighs firmly supported by the pads over their tops. Stabilize this position by performing an isometric seated calf raise to further press your thighs into the pads.

Execution

1. Squeeze your back musculature and drive your elbows down to perform the concentric portion (b).
2. Stop when your personal anatomy organically establishes the bottom position (i.e., you won't be able to move any farther, irrespective of fatigue or load). This is in contrast to focusing on relative bar position to establish your ROM (e.g., bringing the bar down to your clavicles).
3. Reverse the direction for the eccentric portion.

Coaching Tips

- Maintain a roughly vertical torso throughout, by bracing and resisting the urge to flex and extend at the hip throughout.
- Although your back musculature will be in a lengthened position at the end of the eccentric movement, do not stretch the muscle under load.
- Whatever your strength level, you'll always have an opportunity to work on maximally contracting your back musculature. There's a lot going on back there, so use your activation period to practice squeezing different areas using a light load on pull-downs.
- Far too many people use their arms to pull during this exercise, which is especially detrimental during an arm-focused training phase.* To get around this, your focus should be on driving your elbows down to your

*We'll see an exception to this with pull-ups in chapter 10.

sides, using your hands and fingers only as imaginary hooks. To *really* get the feel for this, have a partner place his hands under your elbows and resist you (i.e., he pushes upward) while you perform the concentric movement (i.e., pushing your elbows downward) without weight.

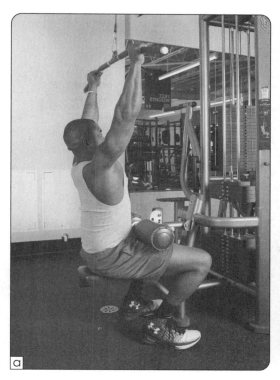
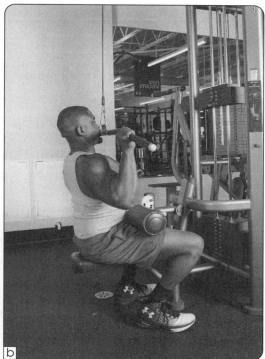

SideBarr

This machine-based exercise is commonly known as a lat pull-down because it engages the large back muscles (i.e., the latissimus dorsi) colloquially known as lats. Unfortunately, most people have never heard of this muscle group, so when they hear the exercise name, their brain turns the sound *lat* into the closest thing it knows. This is why you see people execute by first pulling the bar to their clavicles, and then perform an awkward internal humerus rotation, trying to pseudo-press the bar toward their thighs. As absurd as this seems, the individual is simply performing the exercise that they heard described as *lap pull-downs*. This is all-too-common occurrence serves as a great reminder to be clear with your cueing. Better yet, cue to ignore the bar and execute with your focus on squeezing the back musculature to drive the elbows down. Problem solved.

Foundational Movement 6: Carry

A carry is simply moving your body through space under load, and this might be the biggest compromise of any arm training program. There's a good chance that your forearms and grip strength are already taking a beating on other training days, so there's no need to add to this with carries. Until you get a feel for how fatigued your grip becomes, using wrist straps or at least a hook grip is strongly recommended.

Suitcase Carry

Performing a suitcase (single-arm) carry will allow you to lighten the load on each hand while getting a killer carry session.

Equipment

Dumbbell or kettlebell

Setup

1. Hold the load so that your arm hangs vertically at your side.
2. Stabilize your shoulder and torso before moving.

Execution

1. Walk slowly and work to maintain a tall spine.

Coaching Tips

- Sets are performed for duration or time rather than distance. This allows you to focus on effective form, rather than hurrying to get to the end of your route.

- It is very common to have a limited amount of "runway," resulting in the need for you to turn 180 degrees to reverse the direction. This loaded whole-body rotation is an additional challenge and needs to be balanced between left and right turns, otherwise instinct and habit will always have you turn the same way. To counter this prospective imbalance, we'll employ a trick I learned from power skating: Always face the same wall when making your turns. For example, if you perform a 180-degree right turn during a carry, your next rotation should be to your left (toward the same wall). If your time ends before you need to turn around, be sure to end by facing the same direction in which you started. This may mean that you'll do another 180-degree turn facing the requisite wall, immediately before putting down your load.

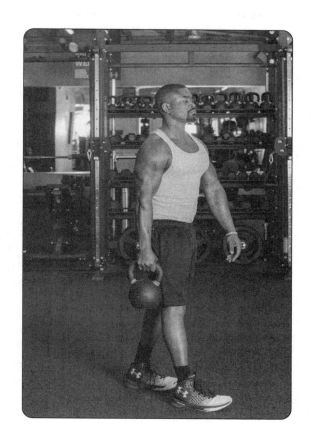

WRAP-UP

We've covered a lot in this chapter, which is only fitting because it addresses the *entire* body. If there was any lingering doubt about training beyond your arms, that archaic thinking should now be gone. Working *with* your body's integrated nature through whole-body training will not only enhance your arm development, but it will also help you to mitigate injury risk and maintain long-term physical function. This begins with bullet proofing your shoulders, which are not only the most mobile joints, but they are directly related to training your biarticular arm muscles. Core strength was next on the list, because its bullet proofing serves as a double win for your arm training and everything else you do in life.

As a bridge between these body parts and the final key target, your traditional warm-up was upgraded to an activation period. In contrast to the traditionally passive obligation, this preparation time will help you dial in your subsequent workout for a more effective muscle stimulus.

The key target of focus was introduced, beginning with the game-changing idea of creating stability for strength. Establishing whole-body tension by screwing your limbs into the ground, bracing, and stabilizing the shoulder will help your nervous system to take the brakes off your strength and thrive during the lift. With enough practice, these components become automatic, which will allow you to benefit from focusing on muscle contraction to move your load. This internal locus of focus targets metabolic growth and really helps you refine your mind–muscle connections.

Lastly, the six foundational movement patterns were introduced along with strategically selected exercises to enhance the performance of each. You'll not only notice the result of their incorporation in your arm musculature, but you'll *feel* it in everyday life.

PART II

The Exercises

Triceps Exercises

Although we're living in a biceps-centric world, it's likely that the triceps muscles actually contribute a greater amount of your arm mass. So, if you're looking for maximum size, triceps training is the best place to start. Recall that the triceps are a biarticular muscle group with the meaty, long head crossing the shoulder joint. We'll take advantage of this through the use the first key (anatomical targeting), by using a variety of pushing and pressing movements, as well as different shoulder positions and grips.

TRICEPS ANATOMICAL TARGETING

The first and most important application of key 1 is to select a variety of exercises based on shoulder position. Recall that the arm muscles are biarticular (crossing both the shoulder and elbow joints), so along with elbow flexion and extension, your shoulder position will affect the feel of contraction and muscle fiber recruitment of each exercise. Triceps exercises fall into three main categories: anterior or elbow up, neutral or posterior, and pressing.

Anterior or elbow up (henceforth referred to as anterior) exercises are performed with the shoulder flexed so that your elbows are in front of you or fully extended overhead. An example would be the overhead cable triceps extension.

Neutral or posterior (henceforth called neutral) exercises occur with the elbows at your sides or behind your torso. An example would be standing cable push-downs.

Pressing consists of exercises that have a combined elbow and shoulder movement (which will be referred to in the drill text as executions). An example is a bench press.

Three Shoulder and Elbow Positions

1. Anterior or elbow up
2. Neutral
3. Pressing

If you're having trouble remembering which exercise falls into which category, you can think of it as where your elbows go, relative to your torso as they extend and flex during each exercise.

FORCE TRANSMISSION— PALMAR AND PINKY GRIPS

A second application for key 1 pertains to the specific points of contact between you and the implement. We are all creatures of habit and tend to grab our implements in the same way during each exercise. By changing up your grip, though, you may experience slightly different muscle fiber recruitment and subsequent feel of contraction. One way to do this is by changing how you grip dumbbells and the cable rope attachment (or V handle attachment) for triceps training.

It is natural to grip a dumbbell at the center of the handle, which means that the friction of our grip across our palm and fingers will transmit the force we exert. This is referred to as a **palmar grip** (figure 4.1*a*). Conversely, rope attachments have a large knob or knot at the end to prevent your grip from slipping. By gripping the rope just above this point and pushing against the knob, much of the force is transmitted across the pinky finger side of your hand. As you might expect, this is called the **pinky grip** (figure 4.1*b*).

As you continually improve your ability to contract different parts of each muscle group, you will come to feel the difference in these two types of grip. This is especially true when you perform dumbbell movements by resting the pinky side of your hand against the end of a dumbbell (as you would the knob on a rope), or when *not* using the knob on the rope (gripping as you would a dumbbell). It really doesn't matter which grip you're using now—the point here is to mix it up to get *all the feels*!

Preview

The specifics of grip and force transmission are also applicable to forearm training and will be discussed in chapter 6.

Force Transmission

1. Palmar
2. Pinky

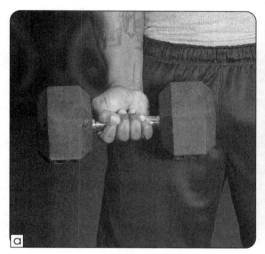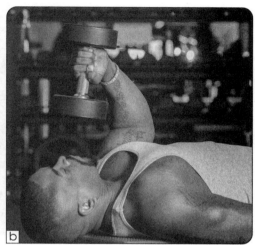

Figure 4.1 (*a*) Palmar grip and (*b*) pinky grip.

TRICEPS EXERCISE DESCRIPTIONS

The most fundamental element of each exercise requires elbow extension during the concentric portion of the movement, so I won't insult you by perseverating that statement. Other general reminders include the following:

- Maintain core stability, stabilize tension (key target 5), optimize stimulus via contraction, and do not throw around excessive weight (key targets 3 and 4).
- For the triceps, you will maintain the palm position or grip that is initially stated, unless otherwise noted.
- Unlike biceps movements, triceps exercises often begin with the eccentric portion of the rep, and this will be explicitly noted where applicable.

Bench Press

It would be pretty hard to write about arm training without discussing the bench press. It fits nicely in our wheelhouse, because in contrast to traditional thinking, it's more of a triceps exercise than a pectoralis exercise. Despite its ubiquity and the fact that an entire day of the week is devoted to its performance (i.e., Monday = international bench press day), the bench press is actually an advanced, very technical movement. Failure to appreciate this has contributed to the decimation of shoulders common to gyms everywhere.

It's important to note that the length of this description does not suggest that this exercise is more important or effective (whatever that would mean). Instead, it reflects the frequent overuse of this advanced movement and subsequent potential for chronic injury. We'll mitigate this to some extent with the Rusin three-way shoulder warm-up, but developing a high level of technical proficiency is still necessary.

We'll detail several components of this exercise, but it's important that you don't try to execute everything at once. Start by picking a couple of cues and practice. If this seems excessively laborious to you, remember that this is a process; even the biggest benchers on the planet are always working on their technique!

Setup

You've seen novices flop around on a bench as they try to move a too heavy of a load—maybe a leg comes up or the bar starts to rotate, until, hopefully, they rack the thing. I've done this myself, but other than the obvious potential for injury risk, it means that we're also leaving a lot of strength potential on the table. One of the biggest game changers for your bench will occur when you develop the skill of maximizing body stability.

The most impactful way to increase stability is through leg drive, which is exactly what it sounds like; you push with your legs to drive your upper back into the bench (figure 4.2). This was my first experience with targeted stability, and although it takes practice, once you nail it, you'll have another oh, my goodness (OMG) moment. You can replicate some of the feel for this by putting your feet up on the bench and performing a glute bridge, trying to force your upper back into the bench. Now work on replicating this with your feet on the ground. I have new clients perform the glute bridge before each set as a tactile cue—a reminder of the feel that they're looking for. When they can replicate this with their feet on the ground, they know that they've achieved full-body stability.

It shouldn't matter if your feet are flat on the ground as long as they are bilaterally symmetrical (i.e., between right and left) and can maximize tension. Also, your legs need a tight core through which they can transmit this powerful stabilizing force, so bracing should be a no-brainer here. Squeezing your shoulder blades and then your lats together will provide upper body stability throughout the entire range of motion (ROM).

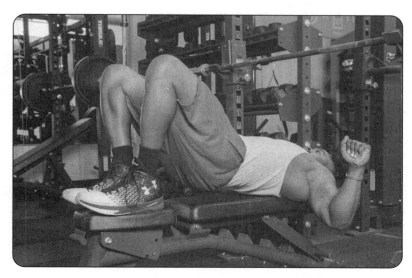

Figure 4.2 To set up the bench press, push with your legs to drive your upper back into the bench.

Grip the bar and wrap your thumbs. Squeeze the bar *hard*, try to externally rotate at the shoulder, and pull the bar apart. The cue for this is that you are trying to bend the bar (table 4.1).

Table 4.1 Bench Press Checklist

Component	Anatomy	Cue
Stability	Legs	Leg drive
	Core tension	Brace
	Retract scapulae	Squeeze shoulder blades together
	Thumb wrap	Thumb
Grip	Squeeze hands	Crush the bar
	Externally rotate arm	Bend the bar
	Abduct arm	Pull the bar apart
Pull-off	Lats	Pull toward your navel

SideBarr: Fix Your Wrist

Along with shoulders and elbows, the other common pain point during the bench press happens at the wrist. The prospective solution begins with targeted anatomy (as is so often the case). The more vertical the downward force from the bar through your hand, wrist, and forearm, the less wrist strain you'll experience. The way to accomplish this is to begin with a traditional wrist-extended position and then *very slightly* flex the wrist. Importantly, your wrists will still be in an extended position; they just won't be *as* extended as they probably were. This places more of the load directly above your forearm as opposed to pushing back on your wrist joint. As a final safety note, you should always feel as though you are in complete control of the bar. If this perception is anything other than 100 percent, you may be flexing your wrist too far, or you may not even need to do so at all. Practice in a squat rack with safety bars, and only employ the wrist flexion tweak with heavier loads once you've developed confidence with this skill using lighter weight.

Once you've just put the effort into creating a stable surface to push through, you don't want to lose it with a traditional lift off of the bar. You want to pull the bar out of the rack toward your navel using your lats, rather than lifting it off with a push. This will ensure that you maintain a tight back and body stability. The best option here is to have a spotter or two set the bar directly over your starting position.

GRIPS AND SHOULDER SPECIFICITY

Grip width has not been mentioned because it comes as a result of first finding your optimal shoulder position. To achieve this, you will use the bottom of the exercise, which is where you end the eccentric part of the rep and begin the concentric part (figure 4.3). Your grip width will be established based on your ability to achieve the most comfortable shoulder position at the bottom, while keeping your forearms vertical. For most people, the bar will land between the lower chest and upper abs, with the elbows abducted roughly 45 degrees away from the body.

If you cannot find a grip and shoulder position without causing discomfort, you may want to replace the bar with dumbbells, replace the bench with push-ups, or eliminate this exercise altogether. You might think that this statement is obvious, but from my own ego-driven experience (and subsequent shoulder issues), the outdated dogma that you have to bench can be a powerful psychological dinosaur.

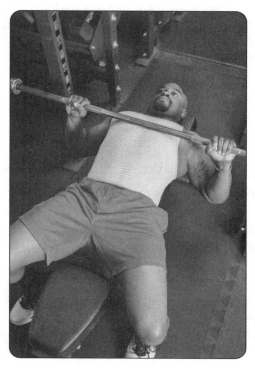

Figure 4.3 Establish your grip width based on the most comfortable shoulder position at the bottom; position your arms at 45 degrees away from the midline of the body.

Lastly, we should all give a nod of thanks to powerlifters for developing these tips. In spite of this transfer, it's also important to note that not every bench press tip is applicable for arm development. Ironically for us, many powerlifting-based suggestions are intended to make the movement easier or reduce the distance that the bar travels, which directly contradicts your goal of stimulating muscle growth.

Decline Extension

The biarticular nature of this exercise allows for a strong recruitment of the long head of the triceps.

Equipment

Dumbbells (or barbell)

Setup

1. Lie on the decline bench with your arms extended and a neutral grip (also known as [aka] palms facing) on the dumbbells (*a*).
2. Maintain a perpendicular arm angle *to your torso* so that they are not completely vertical (relative to the ground), but angled slightly back toward your head. This is the pre-eccentric starting position.

Execution

1. Resist the eccentric part of the rep as your elbows flex (*b*).
2. As you reverse the direction to perform the concentric part, work to resist the instinct of moving your shoulder.
3. Before starting the next eccentric, ensure that your arms are in the starting position, perpendicular to your torso.

Coaching Tip

The common error is allowing the arms to become vertical, which takes much of the tension off the muscle across both joints. For maximum arm development, avoid this instinct to rest and focus on stimulating the muscle.

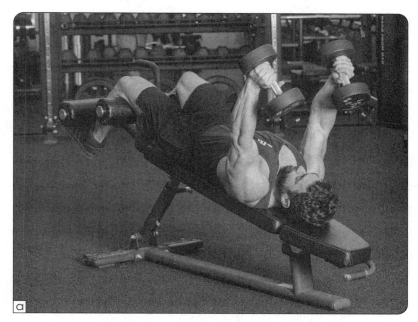

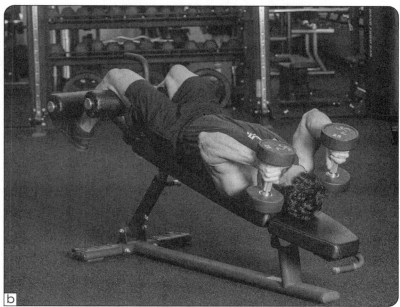

Banded Push-Up

Adding the proper setup to push-ups turns this common exercise into a whole other animal. You may be surprised by how challenging it can be for your core. The use of a resistance band can make this an effective exercise for even seasoned veterans.

Equipment

Elastic resistance and body weight

Setup

1. Wrap the band behind your back under your armpits.
2. Grab the inside of the band in each palm so that it lies between your thumb and fingers. The band should offer the strongest resistance at maximal arm extension.
3. Start from kneeling position and place your palms on the ground slightly wider than shoulder width at the height of your lower chest. This should result in your elbows being approximately 45 degrees abducted (out to your side) at the bottom of the rep.
4. Screw your hands into the ground with external rotation; the cue is that you're trying to make the notch between your biceps and forearms (aka the front of your elbow) face forward. This will usually need to be done with some elbow flexion to take some tension out of the band.
5. With your hands planted, step backward with one leg and drive your toes into the ground for stability.
6. Repeat with the second leg and fire your core (a).

Execution

1. Resist the eccentric part of the rep as your elbows flex and arms extend during descent to the bottom position (b).
2. Reverse the direction to perform the concentric press.

Variations

- Body-weight–only push-ups are an incredibly effective exercise and can be used if a band is unavailable or excessively difficult. The same exercise description applies (with the obvious elimination).
- If a body-weight push-up cannot be executed with proper technique, the movement can be made easier by elevating your hands, for example pushing off of a bench or a wall. This allows you to maintain the full technique, including the essential core and lower body tension.

Coaching Tips

- Wrapping the band under your armpits will minimize the potential for slippage as it loses tension.
- Locking your body with stabilizing tension will ensure that you can drive with maximal force on the push-up.

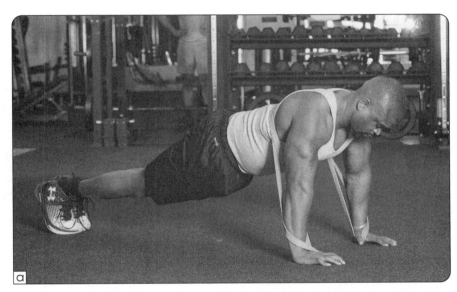

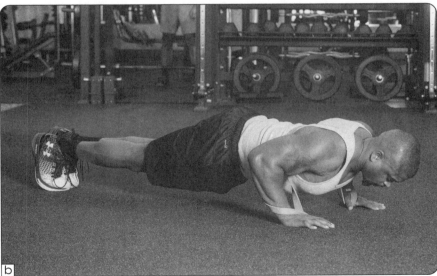

Seated Overhead Extension

Performed with the arm overhead and internally rotated, this exercise provides a novel and powerful feel of contraction.

Equipment

Dumbbell (alternative: cable)

Setup

1. Sit with your hips and knees at 90-degree angles and use both arms to set the dumbbell overhead.
2. The working arm begins at full extension, palm facing forward with the dumbbell directly over the shoulder (*a*). Your nonworking hand and arm can help stabilize your core by grabbing and pressing against your abs.

Execution

While maintaining an approximately vertical arm, perform the eccentric part by resisting the load as your elbow flexes and the dumbbell moves behind your head (*b*).

Coaching Tips

- Although the goal is to maintain a vertical arm, some shoulder movement is natural and inevitable.
- Once you get a pump going, this is an incredibly motivating exercise when performed in front of a mirror. More practically, the mirror provides visual feedback, so you can control the movement and contract the triceps even better.

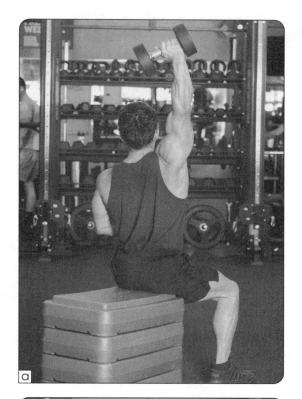

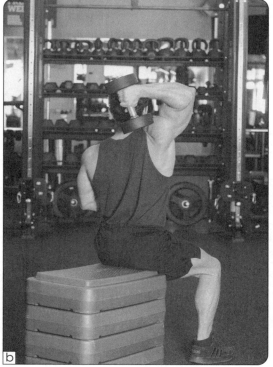

Pit Stain Press

The memorable name of this exercise helps to maintain the cue of keeping your arms locked to your sides, as though you were trying to hide armpit stains in your shirt. Although it's called a press, it's technically an elbow extension exercise that has a strong isometric shoulder extension component.

Equipment

High cable handles (alternative: bands)

Setup

1. Stand at the center of two opposing cable attachments.
2. Grab the handles with an overhand grip and bring your elbows down to your sides (i.e., externally rotate and adduct your humeri). Your arms and forearms will stay between your body and the weight stack throughout. This is the starting position (*a*).

Execution

1. Maintain your shoulder position by keeping your elbows at your sides, as you extend your elbows to bring your hands down to your outer thighs (*b*).
2. Reverse the direction for the eccentric part.

Coaching Tips

- Maintaining the isometric adduction helps to engage the long head of the triceps.
- This can be performed with one arm at a time.

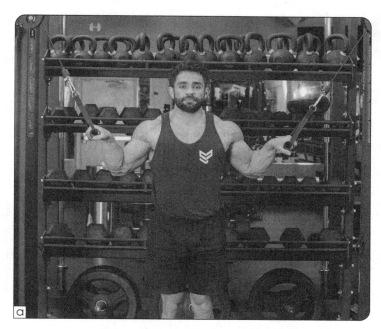

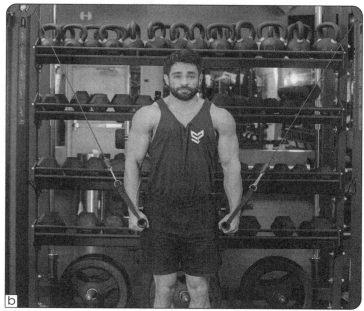

Modified Muscle-Up

This movement is very similar to a traditional cable push-down, but in this case the hands don't move, and your body rotates around them.

Equipment

- Squat rack
- Barbell
- Bench

Setup

1. Anchor the bar in a squat rack at approximately shoulder height.
2. Place the bench close to the rack so you can stand on it in a partial squat, leaning over onto the bar with elbows fully extended and hands pronated on the bar.

Execution

1. Begin the movement with your shoulders over the bar, arms vertical, and toes supporting as much weight as you need on the bench (a).
2. Perform the eccentric part of the rep by resisting as gravity pulls you down, causing elbow flexion and some movement at the shoulder (b).
3. At the bottom of the movement (preconcentric), make sure your knees are flexed behind you with the top of your foot or toes supporting you on the bench.
4. Position your forearms vertically below the bar, which itself will be at approximately chin height.

Coaching Tips

- Although it's designed to isolate the triceps, this movement is more advanced and requires strength throughout your arms, core, upper back, and legs. Start off by performing the top third of the movement and progressively increase your ROM as you get stronger.
- Elbow extension is the primary movement, but enough shoulder flexion happens that this might be thought of as a partial pressing exercise.

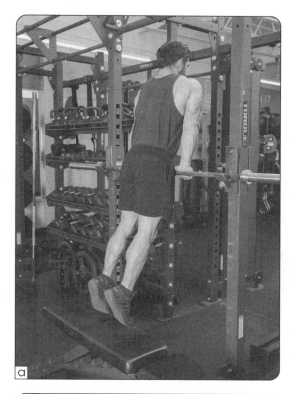

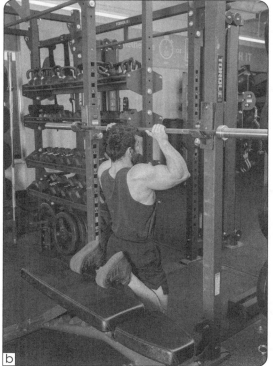

Cable Supinated Extension (One Arm)

This is similar to a dumbbell triceps kickback, but the use of a cable and supinated grip provides tension across the full ROM.

Equipment

High cable handle

Setup

1. Face the weight stack and step laterally just enough that your working arm and forearm are directly in line with the handle.
2. Reach up to grasp the handle with a supinated grip.

Execution

1. Extend your shoulder to bring your elbow down to your side (*a*).
2. Maintain a vertical arm and extend at the elbow, bringing your hand back and down to your outer thigh (*b*).

Coaching Tips

- The supinated grip allows for an unusually strong contraction, although it can become hard to hold the handle as fatigue sets in and your grip strength declines.
- To minimize the impact of grip on execution, use a relatively light weight for this movement.

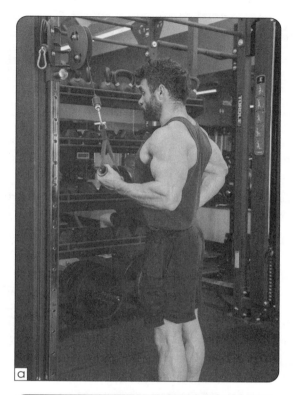

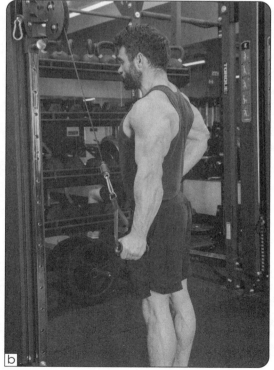

Cross Face Extension (One Arm)

This exercise is the supine (lying faceup) version of the overhead extension. The forward shoulder position and internal rotation of the humerus provide a novel stimulus for the triceps.

Equipment

Low cable handle (alternative: dumbbell)

Setup

1. Lie faceup on a bench, holding a cable handle with a pronated grip and elbow fully extended.
2. Your nonworking arm can help with stabilization by holding your abs.

Execution

1. Start with the cable handle directly over your shoulder, point your elbow out (i.e., internally rotate your humerus), and maintain this vertical arm position throughout (a).
2. Perform the eccentric part by resisting elbow flexion, ending as the handle nearly touches the opposite shoulder (b).

Coaching Tips

- In spite of the name, you are not literally crossing the cable or dumbbell over your face for this exercise.
- If fatigue is causing your core stability or grip strength to suffer, hold off on performing this exercise until your next workout when it can be performed first (when you are fresh).

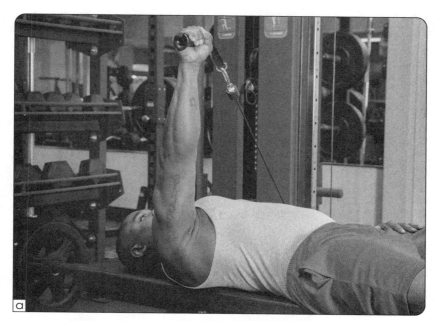

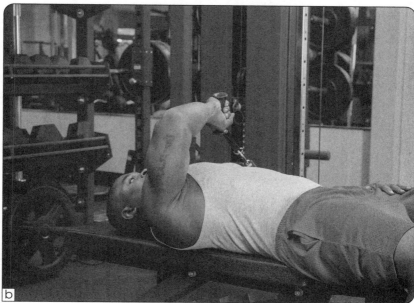

Tiger Bends

This versatile movement may be thought of as an extension-focused push-up.

Equipment

Body weight

Setup

1. Start from kneeling position and place your forearms and palms on the ground shoulder-width apart and parallel to each other.
2. Your hands should be just forward of your shoulders and elbows bent just above 90 degrees (i.e., greatly flexed).

Execution

1. Step backward with one leg and drive your toes into the ground for stability.
2. Repeat with the second leg and fire your core (*a*).
3. Press from the bottom position with a hard, upward drive (*b*).

Coaching Tip

You can elevate your feet if you need to increase the load. Be aware that doing so may change your elbow angle, which is fine as long as it doesn't cause discomfort.

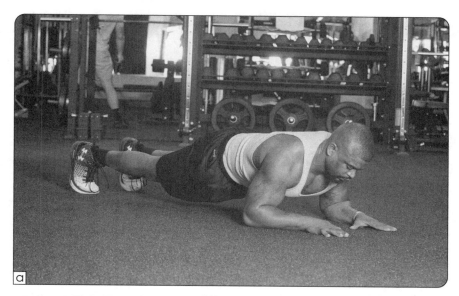

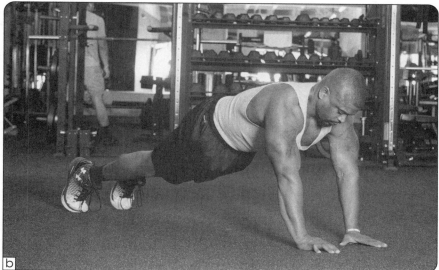

Overhead Rope Extension

This exercise provides maximal tension at full shoulder and elbow flexion.

Equipment

Rope cable attachment (T-handle, etc.)

Setup

1. Face the weight stack to grab the rope with both hands.
2. Turn 180 degrees to face away from the weight stack with your arms overhead.
3. Step forward just enough for the load to develop tension on your triceps, with your elbows flexed (*a*).

Execution

1. Lean forward slightly and adopt a split stance for stability.
2. Maintain your arm position in line with your torso, so that your triceps are next to your ears.
3. Extend at the elbow (*b*).

Coaching Tips

- It is natural to have to readjust your position after the first rep, as long as you're stable for each subsequent rep. If you find that you're still moving around, it is likely that you lack the core or shoulder strength to handle that load and are potentially increasing your risk of injury. Decrease the weight and continue to work on strengthening your core.
- The stretched position across the shoulder and prolonged isometric contraction help to stimulate the long head of the triceps.
- Other cable attachments (such as a T-handle or straight bar attachment) may be used to add variety to the muscle stimulation, although it may be harder to achieve the starting position with them.

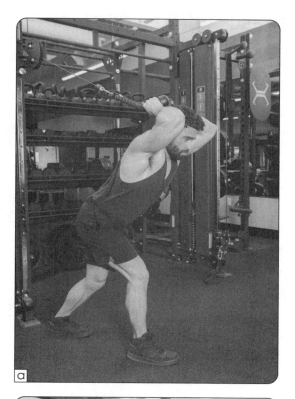

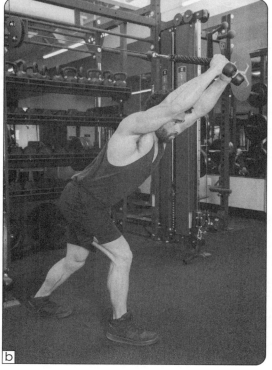

Bench Press Lockouts (aka High Pin Press)

This is an excellent triceps-focused movement, especially for those who have trouble locking out the bench press.

Equipment

- Barbell
- Squat rack

Setup

1. Place the safety bars of your squat rack at a height that will allow you to perform roughly the top third (or less) of the movement.
2. Place the bar at this height as the starting position (*a*).
3. Follow the bench press checklist for your whole-body setup.

Execution

1. Starting from the bottom position, perform the concentric end-range ROM of the bench press (*b*). Reverse the movement for the eccentric part of the rep.
2. The bar should stop dead on the safety bars at the end of each rep (i.e., no bouncing).

Coaching Tips

- Although the reduced ROM will be easier on your shoulders and may allow you to use a heavier load, that is not an excuse to throw around excessive weight. In fact, a heavier load necessitates that you maintain a tight core and lower body stability throughout.
- The exercises to which a pin press can extrapolate is only limited by the use of the bar itself. Stated differently, nearly any barbell movement can employ the use of a partial ROM and dead stop between reps.

Variation

As a variation, hold the full extension (aka lockout) for a three-count.

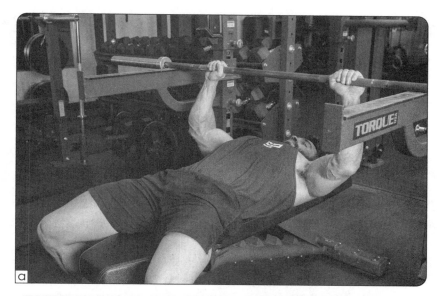

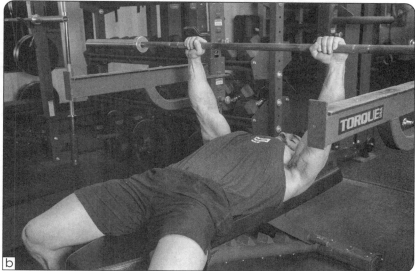

Cable Push-Down

This classic exercise is surprisingly versatile, allowing you to use a variety of shoulder positions and grips to hit the triceps in different ways.

Equipment

High cable T-handle attachment (or rope, V handle, etc.)

Setup

Face the weight stack and grab the T-bar with a pronated grip (*a*).

Execution

1. Bring your elbows down so that they are in line with your torso and maintain this arm position throughout.
2. Lean forward and stagger your stance as needed for balance and stability.
3. Extend your elbows to perform the concentric part of the rep (*b*). Reverse the movement for the eccentric portion.

Coaching Tips

- When trying to maintain this movement as an extension, it is important to fight the instinct to use shoulder involvement.
- Increase your personal awareness of muscle contraction intensity by trying to supinate or pronate at maximal extension. This makes a big difference for some people, so be sure to try this during the warm-up for each workout and see what works best for you.

Variations

- A partial press variant, using some shoulder movement is a viable option provided that this is done so consciously, and not as a result of using too much weight.
- Another variation uses the same elbow extension motion, but with the shoulder maintained in a slightly flexed position at 45 degrees. Keeping your arms just in front of your torso (as opposed to vertical) while you flex and extend the elbow will cause a strong activation of the long head of the triceps. Squeeze your lats and pull your shoulder blades down throughout the entire set for maximal stability and muscle targeting.

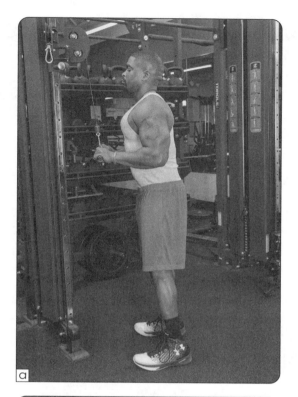

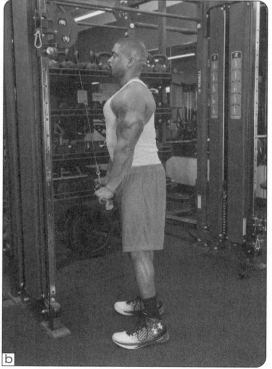

JM Press

Although incredibly effective, this advanced exercise, named after bench press master JM Blakley, uses several technique components. As a result, this movement should be practiced under the verbal guidance of a spotter starting with the lightest bar possible. It might take a few weeks to reach your actual workout load, but the results will be worth it!

Equipment

Barbell (squat rack preferred)

Setup

Lie faceup on the bench, grab the bar with a shoulder-width grip, and extend at the elbows to bring your hands over your shoulders (a).

Execution

1. Perform the eccentric part of the rep by resisting the load as the elbows flex and the shoulders slightly extend, bringing the bar toward your chin.

2. Your elbows will move outward (aka abduct) at roughly a 45-degree angle from the midline of your body.

3. As the bar descends, progressively flex your wrist to create maximal tension at the bottom of the movement (b). This wrist cocking is the difference maker for this exercise. You have to experience it to appreciate it.

4. Ideally, you will let the end of the eccentric part of the rep occur naturally when the forearm hits the biceps, but if not, end the eccentric part when your forearms are nearly horizontal and your elbows are just above chest level.

Coaching Tips

- This exercise should only be done with a spotter or in a squat rack with safety bars. Ideally, you should use both!

- You will feel this in your elbows, and although your tendons will adapt, your muscle will do so more quickly. For this reason, this exercise is used sparingly, giving your tendons a chance to catch up to your strength.

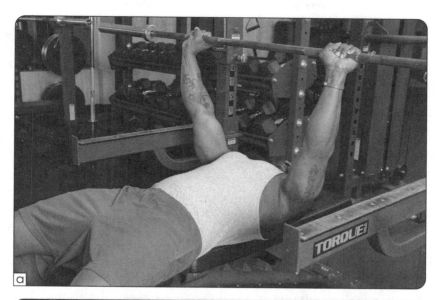

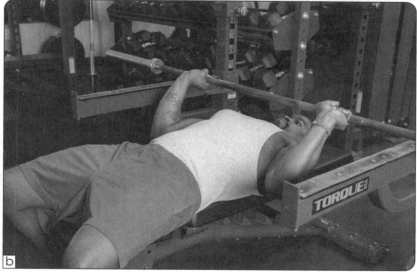

DIPS OVERVIEW

Dips are pressing exercises during which you maintain a fixed hand position and vertical torso and forearms, during which your arms flex and extend behind you.

These exercises are best used to add variety to a program and develop better feel for differences in contraction within the muscle. Because your elbows are behind you throughout the ROM, this can create precarious position for the shoulder. For this reason, dips are best used

- if you have shoulder prehab experience;
- using a limited ROM (two thirds), starting from lockout (i.e., fully extended elbows, pre-eccentric phase); or
- using a relatively light load.

The most common error that you *need* to be aware of happens when the shoulders elevate (toward your ears) and roll forward during the movement. This places a huge strain on the shoulder joint and is a position that should be avoided. To counter this occurrence, use a light weight and focus on keeping your shoulder blades pulled down toward your back pockets. This will organically limit the potentially vulnerable end-range ROM, which is a good thing. Note that increasing ROM might actually feel good in the moment because of the stretch across the shoulder and pectoralis muscles, but this only serves to increase muscle and joint strain without further stimulating your triceps.

Triceps Dips

Equipment

Dip bars

Setup

1. Place your hands on opposite sides of the bars, with your torso between them.
2. Use a bench or step to get into a starting, fully locked-out position (*a*).

Execution

1. With your shoulder blades pulled down, resist the eccentric part of the rep as you descend (*b*).
2. Reverse the movement for the concentric part.

Coaching Tips

- This version of dips usually uses a fixed neutral grip.
- A slight forward lean may be necessary to counterbalance your legs behind you. An excessive forward lean might place more tension on your shoulders and pectoral muscles, at the expense of the triceps that you are trying to target.
- This exercise is particularly taxing on your shoulder stabilizers. Use it only if you've been performing shoulder prehab exercises for several months.
- Your body-weight load can be reduced by placing your feet on a bench behind you. This also removes much of the requirement for core stabilization, so be aware of the huge leap in difficulty when you progress to full body weight.
- Weight can be added by using a weight belt from which a plate is held via a connecting chain.
- Because of the precarious position of the shoulder joint, it is recommended that the full range of motion (i.e., maximal) shoulder extension be avoided. Loaded stretching of a muscle is contraindicated.

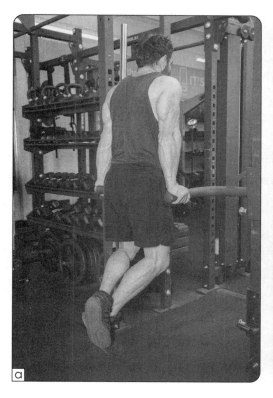 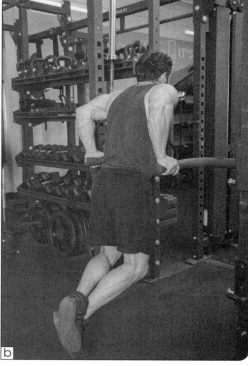

Bench Dips

Equipment

Two training benches

Setup

1. This exercise is performed with your hands pronated on a weight bench positioned behind you.
2. Set your feet up on a second bench in front of you so that your legs are straight (i.e., knees extended) and your hips flexed at roughly 90 degrees (*a*).

Execution

1. Starting at maximal extension (i.e., straight arms), resist as gravity pulls you downward, flexing the elbows and extending the shoulder (*b*).
2. Reverse the direction for the concentric portion of the rep.

Coaching Tips

- Your feet may stay on the ground to decrease the load and subsequent difficulty.
- To make the exercise more challenging, a partner can *gently* add a plate to your lap once your feet are elevated on the bench.

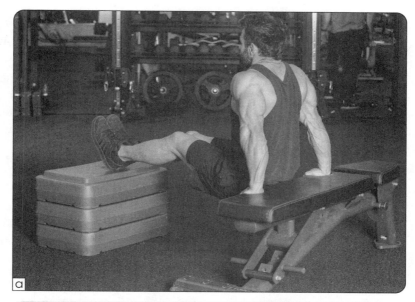

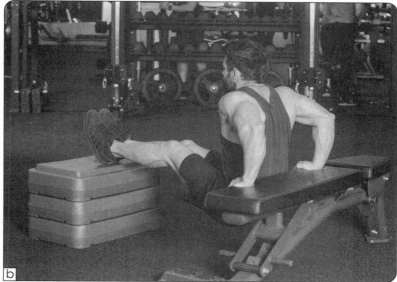

WRAP-UP

The exercises shown in this chapter all require you to target your triceps across a variety of shoulder positions and grips, for *thorough* muscle stimulation. Applying a more detailed setup and execution of the bench press will help you to get more out of this advanced exercise and might just add to your training longevity. Other exercise upgrades, like those for the push-up, will facilitate a stronger mind–muscle connection with your triceps, allowing you to ultimately tap into every fiber for growth.

Biceps Exercises

You might imagine that the current state of biceps training is a good news, bad news situation. The bad news (always start with the bad) is that the biceps are among the most frequently trained muscle groups. The requisite movement (elbow flexion) is basic, and all of the exercises have been done to death. The more we train with these exercises, the less of an opportunity we have for further growth.

The good news is that traditional biceps training has been largely reduced to elbow flexion, which ignores the relatively complex anatomy of this muscle group. This is actually *great* news, because it means that there's a huge amount of untapped potential growth stimulation that your biceps are just begging for.

But don't balk at the idea of applying complex anatomy, because the figurative heavy lifting has been done for you. Your job is simply to apply the concepts and feed your biceps the novel stimulus for growth.

TARGETED BICEPS TRAINING—
SHOULDER POSITION

Similar to the triceps there are three shoulder positions that you will use to anatomically target your biceps training. However, unlike the triceps, for which the neutral and posterior are combined, these positions are distinct for targeted biceps training. Another distinction with biceps is that you do not actively train movement of the shoulder (in contrast to triceps pressing). This is because shoulder flexion is a very weak action for your arm musculature. As a result, most of the load would be handled by the deltoids (anterior shoulder), not your biceps, during this action.

You'll employ exercises with different shoulder positions to create the greatest amount of full range stimulation for your biceps.

Three Shoulder and Elbow Positions

1. Anterior or elbow up
2. Posterior or elbow back
3. Neutral

TARGETED BICEPS TRAINING— WRIST POSITION

Another strategy to target the arms is through the use of three classifications of wrist position and mobility.

1. *Locked grip (also known as [aka] fixed wrist).* The implement does not allow your wrist to rotate.
2. *Unlocked grip (aka open wrist).* The implement allows your wrist to rotate.
3. *Pronated grip (including semipronated).* With this grip, elbow flexion exercises are performed with an overhand or neutral wrist position.

In this chapter we'll discuss the first two grips and save the third for the forearm chapter. Recall that the biceps not only flex the elbow and shoulder, but they also supinate the forearm and wrist. By applying this concept with different exercises, you'll vary the recruitment of your arm musculature to stimulate every fiber.

Locked Grip

The **locked grip** (figure 5.1) happens when an implement forces you to maintain a constant palm and wrist position throughout the entire range of motion, which is best exemplified by a barbell biceps curl. Your wrist cannot rotate (supinate or pronate) as you perform the movement. This allows you to focus mostly on elbow flexion, because you're already locked into a (typically) supinated position.

You may grip cambered bars, like an EZ curl bar using a slightly less supinated grip, but because it is fixed, this is still a locked-grip implement. Note that although you can focus primarily on flexion, you will still probably want to *try* to supinate for maximal biceps activation (i.e., isometrically), in spite of the inability to actually rotate.

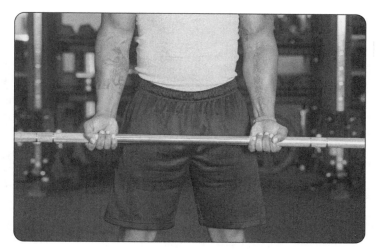

Figure 5.1 Locked grip.

Unlocked Grip

Conversely, when the wrists are able to supinate or pronate throughout the movement, it is called an **unlocked grip** (figure 5.2). Dumbbells and single-handle cable attachments are great examples of implements that provide an unlocked grip, but even a rope attachment qualifies as unlocked, because some rotation can occur. This means that different implements will provide different degrees of freedom for rotation. The result is that you will focus your concentric contraction on both elbow flexion and achieving or maintaining supination when using implements with an unlocked grip.

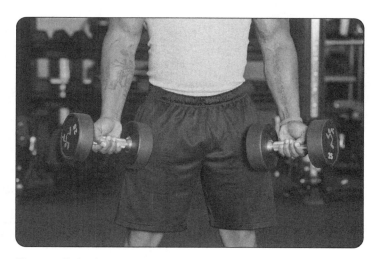

Figure 5.2 Unlocked grip.

Pronated Grip

The first two classifications are based on whether the implement grants you the freedom to rotate your wrist, but the **pronated grip** classification is a little different because it is based on using an overhand (pronated) or neutral (with your palms facing each other; aka semipronated grip) grip, irrespective of implement. Due to their subsequent activation of the brachioradialis muscle, exercises with this grip will be described in chapter 6 (Forearm Exercises).

PERSONALIZED STABILITY— SHOULDER LOCK TECHNIQUE

For biceps training, it turns out that the best stabilization device is your own torso. When you brace your elbows in front of you, they are naturally forced into your torso, effectively locking your arms in place (known as the **shoulder lock technique**, figure 5.3). This creates your own organic "arm blaster," a device that was popularized by Arnold Schwarzenegger in some of his most impressive training pics.

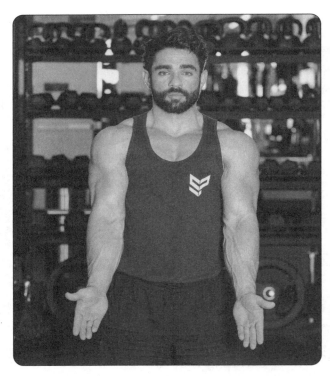

Figure 5.3 Shoulder lock.

By stabilizing the humerus (upper arm bone) in this way, you prevent shoulder movement and eliminate every bit of cheating at this joint. If you're looking to maintain tension on the muscle throughout the full range of motion (ROM) for both time under tension and full-range mechanical loading, this is the easiest way to hit key targets 2 and 4. This also allows you to put more of your focus into isolated muscle contraction (key 5), rather than having to stabilize the load across multiple joints.

As a bonus, it also forces you to naturally stabilize your core—after all, your elbows are digging into you. If, however, you find yourself still leaning back to heave up the load, you're using too much weight and putting yourself at risk for injury.

This technique really shines when you are performing eccentric overload reps, because that is the time that you want the greatest stability and focus on the muscle. As the load increases, your elbow is only stabilized further by being pressed more firmly into your core.

PERSONALIZED GRIP WIDTH— CARRYING ANGLE

Look down at your arms and fully extend your elbows. Although we think of this is as a straight arm, you can see by straightening your fingers that they are not directly in line with your humerus (figure 5.4a). They will be angled away from the body, in line with your forearm. The resulting angle created at your elbow by this difference in alignment between your arm and forearm is known as your **carrying angle**.

It's significant because this natural angle disappears as you flex the elbow, so that your forearm and humerus become aligned (at the top of a curl, for example, figure 5.4b). This means that *the distance between your hands naturally changes from the bottom to the top of a curl*, which can become challenging with locked-grip exercises. The natural change in distance between hand positions when the elbow is fully extended (bottom) and fully flexed (top), is called the **grip delta**. Because the size of the carrying angle differs between individuals, the grip delta can be *huge* in some people. This might result in elbow pain when performing a locked movement, especially when using a grip width that is traditionally selected using fully extended elbows (e.g., picking up a bar from the ground, or from a rack at roughly waist height).

Further, if you're executing curls using a wide grip based on carrying angle (at the bottom of the movement), you can end up with an awkward ineffectual flexed-end ROM, rather than a tight, focused squeeze. In this situation, your body is often just trying to figure out what it's supposed to do, rather than contracting your arm musculature. After some investigation, it turns out that this is a surprisingly common phenomenon.

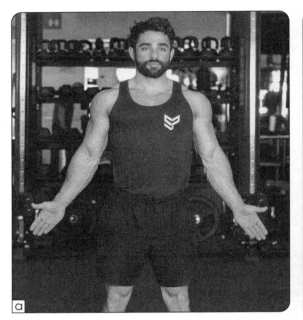
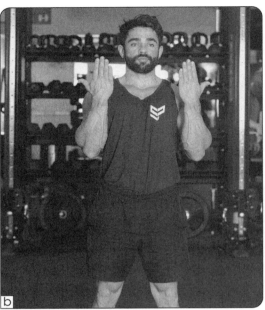

Figure 5.4 (*a*) Straight arms and (*b*) flexed arms.

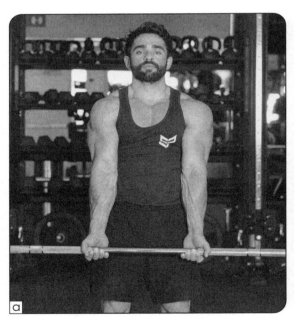
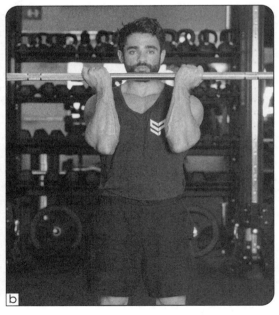

Figure 5.5 (*a*) Establishing hand spacing with shoulder lock and (*b*) applying hand spacing.

The solution to this is to choose your grip based on your hand spacing at the peak contracted position. This works especially well with the shoulder lock technique, which is naturally going to result in a narrower grip (figure 5.5a). Your flexion will likely be stronger, and you should feel a better squeeze of the biceps at peak ROM (i.e., maximal elbow flexion grip (figure 5.5b).

Although this anatomically targeted upgrade can't eliminate the grip delta, you'll probably find it easier to supinate at full extension with a slightly narrower grip, compared to the more common situation (i.e., an excessively wide top portion of the movement). If you find that this creates the opposite problem, in that your fully extended position is awkwardly narrow, you can choose a slightly wider grip and progressively work on extended supination.

Importantly, there's no single grip width that's correct or incorrect; it's simply important to be aware of all of the tools available for your training arsenal. Some people find this one change makes a huge difference, so be sure to play with different grip widths and the resulting intensity of contraction throughout each exercise!

CURL EXERCISES

Although we're focused on the relatively simple motion of elbow flexion, recall that the biceps cross the shoulder joint, which is the most mobile joint in the body. This gives us an incredible variety of opportunities to apply key 1 by changing joint angles in our efforts to tap the growth potential of every muscle fiber. For example, if your shoulder is flexed so that you're in the elbow-up position, this means that the biceps are slightly shorter across the shoulder (figure 5.6a). Conversely, when your arm is behind your torso (elbow back), as it is for incline dumbbell curls, your biceps will be in a more a lengthened position (figure 5.6b). In turn, this lengthened position changes the feel of the contraction and fiber recruitment.

It is with this level of anatomical specificity that these exercises have been selected to optimize your arm development. By providing locked and unlocked grip variations, different shoulder positions, and implement choices, you'll experience a variety of resistances across the ROM to reach even the most stubborn fiber.

Coaching tips and descriptions are provided along with the imagery for each elbow flexion exercise. Unless otherwise noted, the exercise description will end immediately prior to the concentric phase, which you can universally imagine as "squeeze your biceps to flex your elbow and supinate," after which you return to the starting position via the eccentric phase (by definition).

We want you to get to lifting rather than reading about it, so to further eliminate redundancy, statements such as brace your core, create stabilizing tension throughout your body, maintain shoulder position, keep your wrists straight, don't be stupid by throwing weights around, and so on, are implied for each exercise.

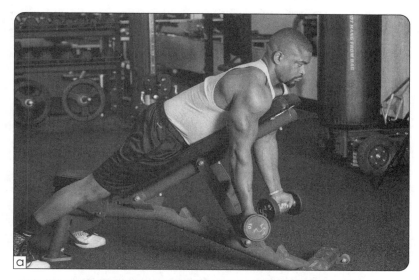

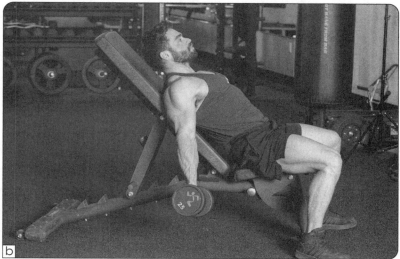

Figure 5.6   (*a*) Elbow up and (*b*) elbow back.

Preacher Curl

This exercise provides stability for the arm and shoulder, which allows you to focus on contracting the biceps.

Equipment

Barbell (alternative: dumbbells or machine)

Setup

1. Anchor your arms fully against the pad, with your armpits on the top of the pad (*a*).
2. Unless you have a partner handing you the weight, you will need to begin this exercise with the eccentric contraction.

Execution

1. Dig your elbows into the pad and create tension in your back to decrease the risk of your shoulders rounding forward throughout the movement.
2. With stabilizing tension being generated, resist the eccentric contraction as your elbows extend. Stop in a bottom position that allows you to maintain tension on the muscle (*b*). This is not necessarily full elbow extension for everyone.
3. Reverse the movement for the concentric portion, stopping the movement before you lose tension on the muscle.

Coaching Tips

- Recall that this exercise can have an extreme force delta, with maximal loading at the bottom (fully extended) portion of the ROM. Although you can experience a great contraction with the muscle lengthened, this should not turn into loaded stretching. Use an ROM specific to your abilities and only work on biceps flexibility when you're *not* loaded.
- Maximal flexion is also contraindicated because there is no tension on the muscle through the top ROM, so skip approximately the final 15 degrees. People love to rest in this tension-free dead zone, so fight your instinct and focus on the task of stimulating your muscle.
- Maintain full arm contact with the bench throughout the full ROM. Your shoulder should not move.
- There's no need to use a seat. Supporting your body weight with your arms and legs, by partially squatting, will allow you to drive your arms into the pad for greater stability.
- The lengthened position of the muscle and potentially rounded forward shoulder could result in mild shoulder strain. If you feel any discomfort in the front of your shoulder, stop the exercise.

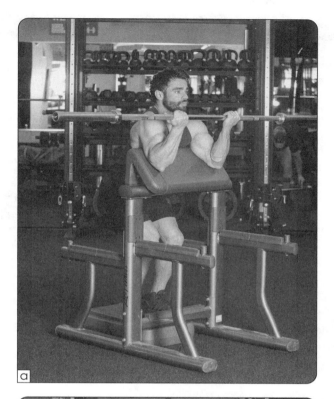

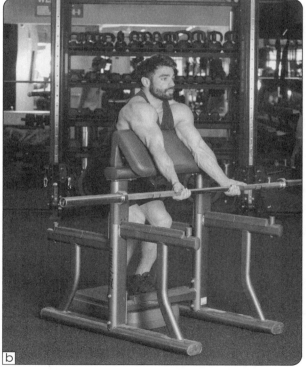

Caulfield Curl

Introduced to me by strength coach Scott Caulfield, this innovative variation of a preacher curl combines a stable arm position with an unusually high frontal arm position. The resulting intensity of the contraction is hard to replicate.

Equipment

Low cable attachment (alternative: band)

Setup

1. Sit facing the weight stack with your hips flexed at roughly 45 degrees relative to your torso. This means that your knees will be close to your torso and serve as a support for your arms as you curl (*a*).
2. Grasp the attachment, such as a T-bar or D-handles.
3. Lean forward and place your elbows on your knees as support.

Execution

1. Beginning at full extension, flex your elbow to curl the load (*b*).
2. Maintain hip and shoulder angle throughout the set.
3. Reverse direction for the eccentric portion.

Coaching Tip

This elbows-up position is similar to a preacher curl but provides a more consistent level of tension throughout the full ROM.

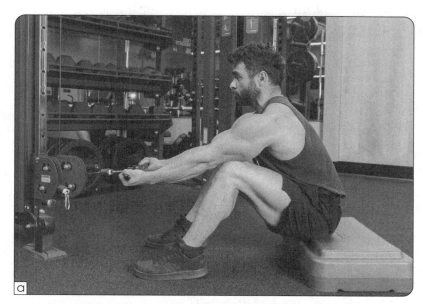

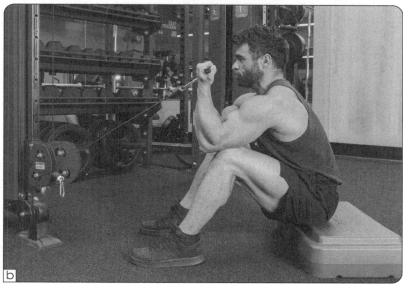

Spider Curl (aka Prone Biceps Curl)

A stable frontal shoulder position provides versatility and allows you to focus on contractions with the biceps in a doubly shortened position.

Equipment

Dumbbells (or barbell)

Setup

Grasp your dumbbells and lie face down on a bench that has been inclined enough to allow you to reach full extension with your arms roughly perpendicular to your torso (a).

Execution

1. Beginning at full extension, flex your elbow to curl the load (b).
2. You should have enough clearance that your implements do not touch the ground throughout the set.

Coaching Tips

- Create whole-body tension by pressing your feet into the ground. Although the key of stabilizing tension applies to every exercise, the often-omitted leg drive is especially helpful here.
- If using a barbell, you will likely need to have a partner assist you in order to set up safely.

Variations

- Experiment with different angles of bench and subsequent shoulder position. Although you want to maintain tension across the full ROM, this exercise affords some versatility with regard to starting shoulder position and final elbow position (peak flexion).
- Increase your amount shoulder flexion (starting with your arms a little closer to your head) to create a shorter muscle length throughout which you contract.
- Start with your shoulder flexed, only to extend it (bring your arm backward) toward your waist as you flex the elbow.

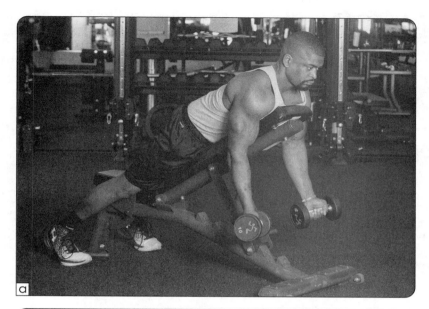

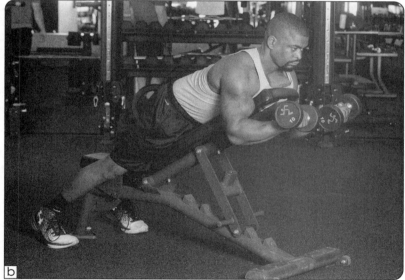

Behind-the-Back Standing Cable Curl

Triple tension across the shoulder, elbow, and wrist makes this exercise a fantastic addition to your training arsenal.

Equipment

Low cable attachment and single handle (e.g., D-handle; alternative: band)

Setup

1. Grip a single handle and face away from the weight stack.
2. Step away from the load until there is tension on your arm at maximal extension, with your hand at or just behind your hip (*a*).
3. Take a split stance for stability.

Execution

1. Beginning at full extension, flex your elbow to curl the load while maintaining shoulder position (*b*).
2. Maintain tension on the biceps and forearm throughout the set.

Coaching Tips

- This exercise offers resistance on your biceps throughout the full ROM, as well as a little isometric resistance across the shoulder and wrist.
- Having the elbow slightly behind you so that the biceps are in a slightly lengthened position at the shoulder allows for an intense peak contraction.
- Experiment with swapping the leg position on the side of the working arm. For example, if you naturally perform sets with this leg in front, try performing the exercise with it as the rear leg.

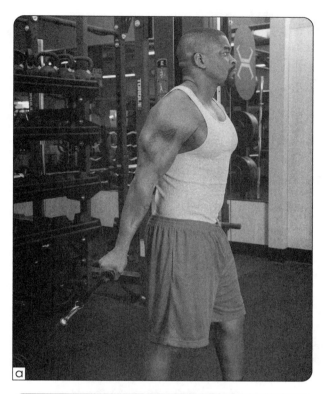

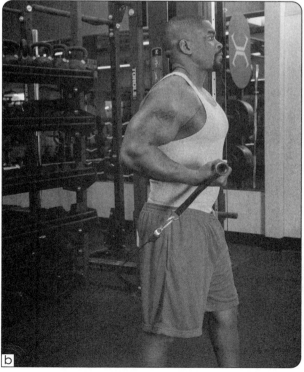

Clayton Curl

This unusual three-phase exercise combines different elbow and shoulder positions for a powerful eccentric movement.

Equipment

Low cable attachment

Setup

1. This is a three-phase exercise that starts by adopting a split stance with the low cable attachment behind you.
2. The hand on the side of your back leg starts at—or just behind—your hip (*a*).

Execution

1. Imagine a pin connecting your elbow to the side of the body and maintain this position as you flex the elbow to peak contraction (*b*).
2. For the eccentric phase, you can imagine pushing your hand down just forward of your hip, moving toward your front pocket (*c*).
3. Push your elbow forward slightly as your hand moves down an imaginary vertical line.
4. At full extension, allow your hand to return to the starting position behind you, to perform another rep.

Coaching Tips

- This is a great novel contraction on the eccentric phase, as both the elbow and shoulder move.
- The nature of this exercise requires that a light load be used, but that does not diminish its effectiveness.

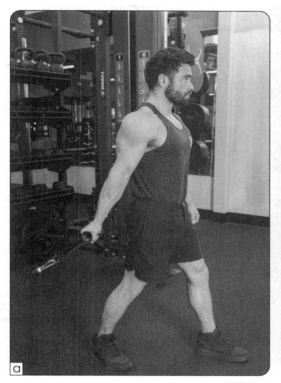

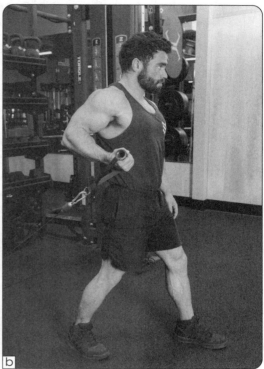

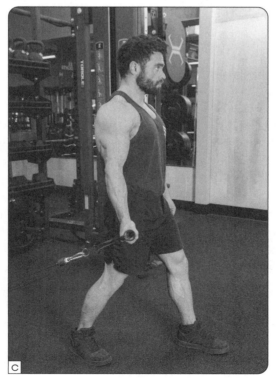

Nilsson Curl (aka Chin-Up Curl)

Similar to a chin-up, this exercise locks your forearms in place and places all of the emphasis on your biceps.

Equipment

- Squat rack
- Two barbells

Setup

1. Set your safety bars just above shoulder height in a squat rack and place a barbell on them at the back of the rack against the cage.
2. Set your second barbell up so that it rests on the barbell supports (often known as J-cups or J-hooks) above the first barbell. The distance between bars is determined by the length of your forearm.
3. Grip the top bar and rest your elbows against the bottom bar, locking your forearms in place (*a*).

Execution

1. The movement is similar to a chin-up with your forearm braced against the lower bar.
2. From a hanging position under the bars, flex your elbows by squeezing your biceps (*b*).
3. Due to the inherent difficulty, the initial set up allows you to use your legs to provide as much assistance as necessary.

Coaching Tips

- As you become stronger, you will not need the support of your lower body to perform this movement, in which case your initial setup can be higher in the rack.
- This exercise is unusual in that the forearm and wrist are locked in position, while the body moves around the elbow joint.
- Stabilize your shoulders throughout this movement so they do not roll forward, which may happen to provide the illusion of getting closer to the bar at the top. This shoulder cheat will cause excessive, undesirable stress on the biceps tendon across the shoulder.
- As your brain and muscle learn to coordinate to better perform this exercise, you may want to deload much of the concentric portion with your legs and use a partial ROM throughout.

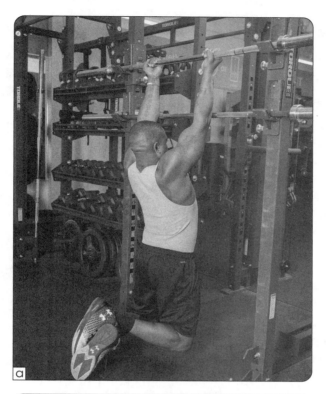

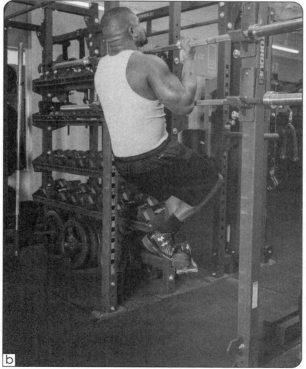

Concentration Curl

Once a punchline demonstrating the impotence of isolation exercises, the concentration curl has emerged from the ashes as the thinking man's curl.

Equipment

Dumbbell (or low cable)

Setup

1. Sit on a bench with your knees and ankles bent at 90 degrees.
2. Rest the back of your working arm on the inside of your thigh and place your nonworking hand on your other knee for support (*a*).

Execution

1. Squeeze your arm to flex the elbow.
2. Reverse the direction for the eccentric portion (*b*).
3. Maintain tension across the full ROM; do not rest at the top or bottom.

Coaching Tips

- It's hard to beat the level of peak contraction that this classic exercise allows. This is due to the combination of arm stability, elbow-up (aka shoulder-flexed) position, and cross-body movement (i.e., internally rotated humerus) unique to this exercise.
- Be sure to stare intently at your working biceps and imagine them becoming as big as the Austrian Alps!

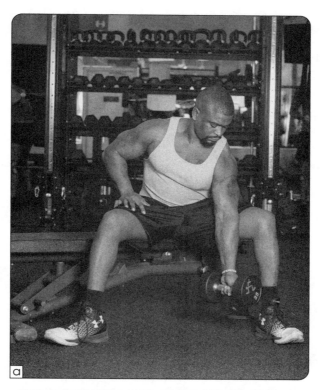

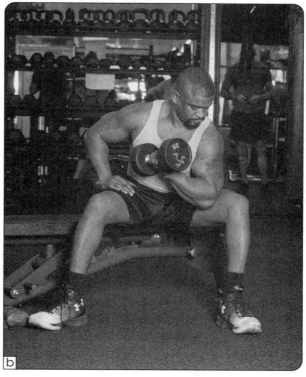

Harski Hammer Curl

This innovative exercise uses a barbell to create the feel of a cross-body dumbbell curl. Better yet, elastic resistance allows you to maintain tension, even at maximal ROM.

Equipment

- Light barbell (mace bell preferred)
- Elastic resistance band

Setup

1. One hand serves as support for the immobile end of the barbell, while the hand of the working arm is supinated, gripping the other end of the bar (*a*).
2. The elastic resistance is looped over the end of the bar with the hand of the working arm and is anchored low and in front of you so that it produces maximal tension (i.e., it has the greatest amount of stretch) at the top of your flexed ROM.
3. For example, if you were standing in the center of an imaginary clock face (or compass) on the ground, the anchor would be at the 1:30 position for your working right arm (alternative: NE position on a compass).
4. The support arm is locked with its hand holding the immobile end of the bell.

Execution

1. Curl the bar with the working arm, slightly crossing the bar toward the center of your body (*b*). As a cue, the hand of your working arm will complete the concentric portion near the center of your chest.
2. Reverse the motion for the eccentric portion.

Coaching Tips

- This exercise is unusual in that it begins fully extended at your carrying angle and the elbow flexes across the body.
- As the barbell or mace bell load progressively decreases as you flex your elbow, the band tension increases to give you tension across the full ROM.
- For safety, always maintain a small amount of tension in the band at its shortest length. This will minimize the risk of having it become lax and slip off the bar.

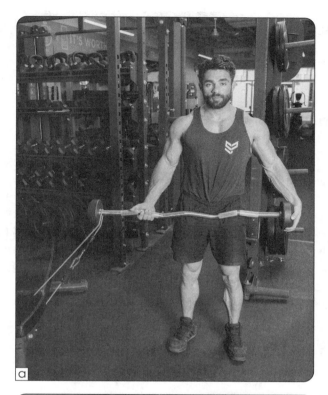

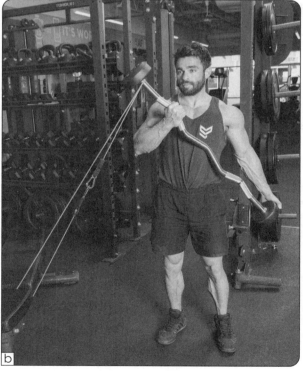

Cable Flex Curl (aka Double Biceps Pose)

If you've ever wanted to stare at yourself in a mirror while maximally contracting your biceps against a load (and let's face it, *you have*), this is the exercise for you.

Equipment

Two opposing high-cable attachments

Setup

1. This exercise replicates your first intentional biceps contraction, which likely happened as a response to the verbal encouragement of "Make a muscle!" You may be more familiar with the bodybuilding parlance and refer to it as the double biceps pose.

2. Grab the handle of each opposing high-cable attachment and center yourself between the weight stacks (*a*).

3. Each arm should be roughly parallel to the ground throughout the movements.

Execution

1. Squeeze your biceps to flex your arms (*b*).

2. Reverse the direction for the eccentric portion.

Coaching Tips

- The high frontal shoulder position and external rotation of the arm provides a strong novel stimulus from the contraction.

- Although it's possible to perform a similar high-elbow cable movement while facing the weight stack, the resulting instability makes it a less effective stimulus.

- By using the opposing handles as counterweights, you're effectively adding to the stability of this exercise. It also makes it very hard to cheat during this exercise.

- Performing this exercise in front of a mirror is not only incredibly motivating, but it allows you to visually focus on the contraction.

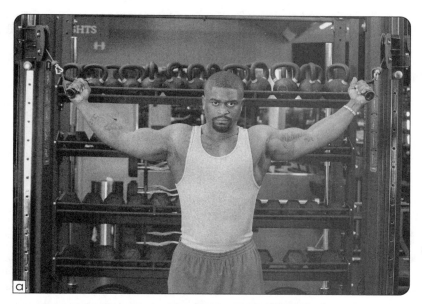

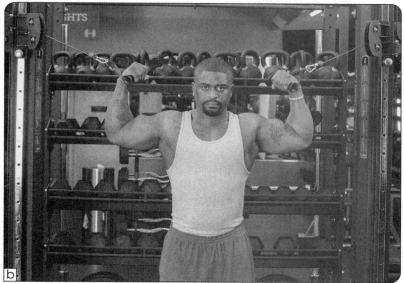

Barbell Curl

This is probably the most basic form of biceps exercise and a great opportunity to employ the shoulder lock technique.

Equipment

Barbell (straight or EZ curl)

Setup

1. Establish whether you are using the shoulder lock technique. If you are, you'll need to set your grip up with your hands closer together on the bar.
2. After including the grip adjustment for shoulder lock, determine your final grip width based on carrying angle, or its omission.
3. Grab the bar with a supinated grip.
4. If you are using the shoulder lock, flex your shoulders slightly to bring your arms forward and rest your arms against your core (*a*). Otherwise your arms can stay at your sides.

Execution

1. Brace your core and contract your biceps to curl the bar (*b*).
2. Your elbows should not move unless you're intentionally experimenting with the feel of contraction (see the first coaching tip that follows).
3. Resist the load as you reverse the direction for the eccentric portion.

Coaching Tips

- During your warm-up (or when using a light load) you can experiment with the peak contraction (i.e., maximal flexion) by holding this position for just a moment before pushing your elbows slightly forward for a second, and then performing the eccentric portion. This elbow push shortens the biceps across the shoulder joint, which provides a slightly different contractile stimulus to the muscle.
- The elbow push should not be used to take tension off of the biceps. It is used to stimulate, not serve as a rest.
- To ensure that you're not cheating by heaving the bar up with your back (aka the lower back killer), use a split stance or brace yourself against a solid vertical surface, like a pole or wall.

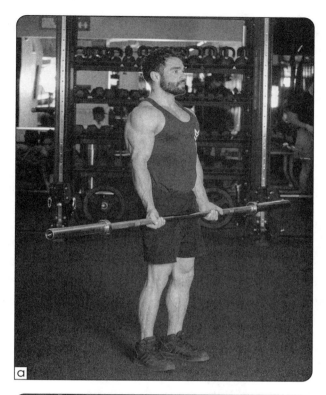

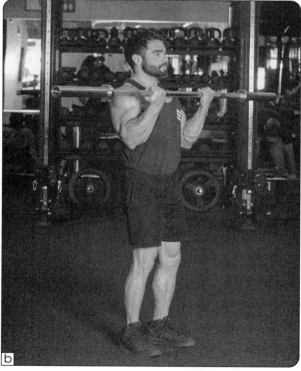

Drag Curl

This exercise is a curl with a seemingly innocuous neutral shoulder position that morphs into an artificially induced posterior shoulder position. This exercise must be experienced to be fully appreciated.

Equipment

Barbell or Smith machine

Setup

This movement is similar to a standard barbell curl that uses a completely vertical bar path (*a*).

Execution

1. Flex your elbows and drag the bar up your torso (i.e., maintain close proximity of the bar to your thighs and torso throughout the movement (*b*).
2. You do not need to make the bar actually contact your body, provided that the bar movement path is vertical.
3. Allow your elbows to naturally drive back and up as you flex at the elbow.

Coaching Tips

- This is an unusually intense contraction as your biceps flex at the elbow while simultaneously lengthening across the shoulder. For this reason, a lighter weight is used than would be for standard barbell curls.
- A Smith machine is a great optional implement, because it locks you into a vertical track and can be a great way to learn this counterintuitive bar path.

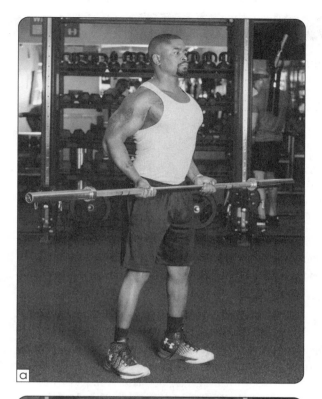

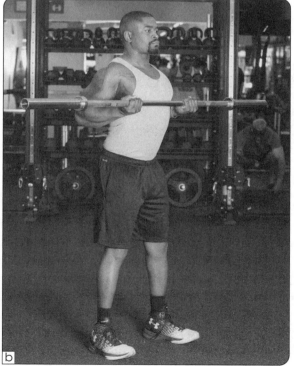

Incline Curl

The incline curl is a biceps exercise that uses the rarely achieved posterior shoulder position.

Equipment

Dumbbells (alternative: cable)

Setup

1. Grab the dumbbells and sit back on an incline bench.
2. Let your arms hang vertically (*a*).

Execution

1. Maintain this arm position as you flex at the elbow (*b*).
2. Reverse the movement for the eccentric portion, ending before you lose resistance at the bottom.

Coaching Tips

- This exercise provides resistance through full ROM, as long as you avoid the instinct to let your arms rest at the bottom This is often done because we like the feeling of a stretch, but the tension in the bottom position should not be confused with resistance. Further, loaded stretching is contraindicated.
- The natural lengthened position of the biceps at the shoulder provides an intense arm contraction.

Variation: Single-Arm Low-Cable Curl

1. Attach a single handle to a low a cable apparatus.
2. Face the bench away from the weight stack and grab the handle.

Coaching Tips

- Note that rather than gravity pulling your arms down, the cable will actually pull your arm *back*.
- This exercise is performed only for chasing the feel of a different muscle contraction. This means that a very light load should be used, with an intense focus on contracting the muscle.
- You may also need to focus on pushing your elbow forward slightly (to create a vertical arm) to resist the cable from pulling you back. This additional requirement adds a little more tension to the biceps and also contributes to the need of reducing the weight.
- This exaggerated lengthening of the biceps might feel great at first, but loaded stretching of the biceps and shoulder are potentially injurious and therefore contraindicated.

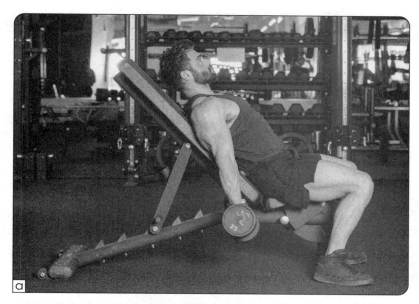

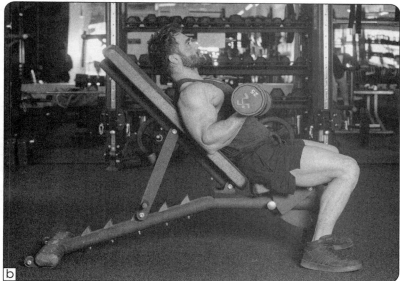

Low-Cable Cross-Body Curl

This exercise provides a great cross-body contraction, but you should be aware that it requires a large amount of shoulder stability.

Equipment

Two opposing low-cable attachments

Setup

1. Grab the handle of each opposing low-cable attachment and center yourself between the weight stacks.
2. Your palms should be facing forward, and your arms abducted at 45 degrees from your torso (i.e., from the front, you should look like a peace symbol) (*a*).

Execution

1. As you flex at the elbow, bringing your hands in front of you, just as they do with any other curl (*b*).
2. Finish the concentric action when your hands nearly touch each pectoralis muscle.

Coaching Tip

You may feel the instinct to cheat the movement by pushing your elbows forward as you flex the elbow. Be sure to minimize this shoulder flexion to avoid turning this into a deltoid exercise at the expense of biceps stimulation.

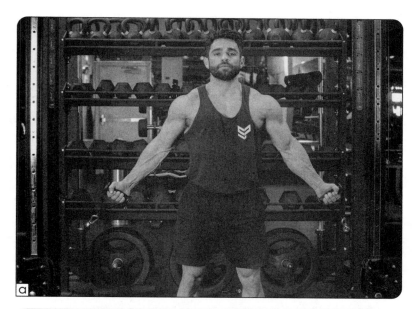

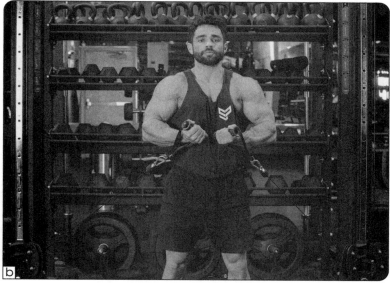

WRAP-UP

We've explored so much anatomical opportunity for growth in this chapter, you might already be feeling a pump in your biceps. You've seen how changing both shoulder angle and wrist rotation can affect your biceps activation rather than causing mere elbow flexion. Further, applying the shoulder lock technique and grip delta allow you to use your own personalized anatomy for stimulating the target musculature. Using different movements and implements will ensure that you can access every fiber, and you'll get better with every rep.

Forearm Exercises

If you were to ask me why we're spending a whole chapter on forearms, I'd answer: "Because they're listed in the title of the book." But when I was done laughing at my *hilarious* joke, I'd offer this sobering reality: "Forearms are the most visible naked muscle group you have." As a bonus, developing your grip strength will make you stronger in every other exercise. Taken together, the exercises in this section help you to perform and to make an impression. If you need more convincing, as I did, consider the following.

Perhaps the best way to pay homage to someone who has inspired your training is to name an exercise after him. This has never been more applicable than with strength coach and gym owner Matt Wenning. He is an elite powerlifter who has achieved the inhuman milestone of a 1,000-pound (453 kg) squat during which he stated that he could feel his femurs bow (pause for a moment and let that sink in). But let's skip all of those achievements (and contributions to this work) and name a forearm isolation exercise after him: Wenning wrist flicks.

The reason he deserves this tremendous honor can literally be felt when you shake his hand; it's surprisingly muscular. Now you may have felt large hands, or thick hands, but it's unlikely that you've ever felt a *muscular* hand. This adds another exclamation point to his already imposing physique. It also provides another reason for you to train forearms and grip when you're trying to make an impression: a firm handshake might imply confidence, but meaty forearms and a strong handshake actively *demonstrate power*.

ANATOMICAL TARGETS

There are dozens of muscles and joints in the hand and forearm, and the amount of available detailed information is staggering. As I started to go down the anatomical rabbit hole, a lesson from the legendary Bruce Lee came to mind. Although he had studied these same muscles and joints, he omitted their inclusion in his opus *The Tao of Jeet Kune Do*. The reason was that the application of such minutiae was limited, which necessitated focus on broader, more practical elements. And so it is with this work. We'll target the brachioradialis muscle and forearm flexors to help you develop the most naked of all muscle groups and make a powerful impression.

Consistent with most limb muscles, many of the forearm muscles are biarticular. This means that we can anatomically target forearm training by changing elbow, wrist, or hand position during different exercises. For the sake of simplicity, it will suffice for you to merely be aware of that fact and apply it on an as-needed basis. The following exercises will be an overview from which you can vary at your discretion.

As with triceps training (chapter 4), using a rope or dumbbell allows you to vary your points of contact through which you transmit force to the implement (and vice versa). Changing your grip from a palmar grip (see figure 4.1a on page 87) and resting the index finger and thumb side of your hand against the implement (an **index and thumb grip**) can alter the feel and muscle activation of the exercise.

Force Transmission

1. Palmar
2. Index and thumb

If you're new to flexion exercises performed with a neutral or pronated grip, it's important to maintain awareness of the amount of work and degree of stretch you experience across the brachioradialis throughout your training program. This is especially important if you're new to incorporating pull-ups, which can be very taxing on the brachioradialis—particularly at the fully stretched bottom position.

Similarly, although grip training can provide a massive upgrade for your forearm mass and overall strength, hold off on performing too much of this work as you start a new program. The novel stimulus may be enough to fatigue your grip even without specifically training it, which could negatively affect the rest of your lifts. As your grip strength and endurance naturally improve, you can slowly add in more specific work to accelerate these processes.

Things to Remember

- As a general reminder, a palms-facing grip is also known as a neutral, semipronated, or semisupinated grip.
- Although you'll still target your attentional focus on the muscle, you don't want to waste energy trying to isolate small muscles to contract. You're better off squeezing the general arm musculature to move the load and stimulate the target muscles organically.
- Perform grip training at the end of your workout. You won't be able to do anything other than body-weight work if you can't grab the weight!

Thick-Grip Training

This isn't an exercise itself but rather a simple way to improve grip and forearm development without major program changes. The trick is to enlarge the diameter of any implement, like a dumbbell or barbell, which makes it harder to hold and perform the exercise (see the below image of a thick-grip dumbbell curl). The reason you would do this is to change the recruitment of the primary muscles (Krings et al. 2019) and increase grip strength and forearm size. The additional benefit is that you will feel much stronger on subsequent sets with a normal-diameter grip.

The best way to employ thick-grip training is to use a thick bar or by using attachments specifically intended for this purpose. If you don't have access to either of these, you can use anything that will fit snugly over your implement. In the past, I've used dense foam pipe coverings and tightly wrapped hand towels, which are low cost and widely available.

The simplest implementation is to perform a single warm-up set of each exercise with a thick grip. Not only will this help to develop your grip strength and forearm mass, but your work sets will feel far more locked in.

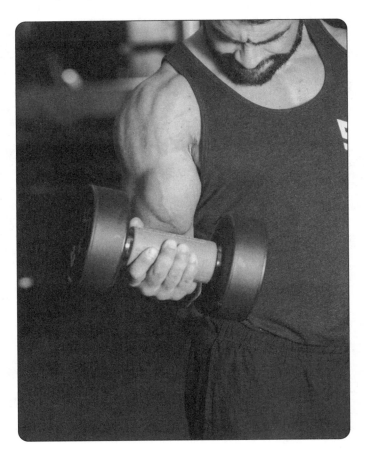

Pronated Barbell Curl

This classic flexion exercise targets the brachioradialis muscle, which you might recognize as the "teardrop" of the arm. Teardrop is a common name for the medial thigh muscle above the knee.

Equipment

Barbell

Setup

Grasp the bar with an overhand grip with your hands approximately shoulder-width apart (*a*).

Execution

1. Brace and squeeze your arm musculature to flex the elbow (i.e., curl the bar) (*b*).
2. Maintain a straight wrist and vertical arm position throughout.

Coaching Tips

- During your warm-up (or when using a light load), you can experiment with a false grip by keeping your thumb over the top of the bar with the rest of your fingers.
- Eliminating the thumb support during this movement changes the feel of the contraction and places a greater load on your finger-specific grip.
- You should not be at risk of dropping the bar at any point.

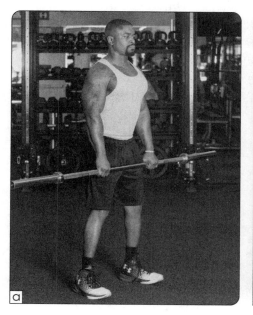
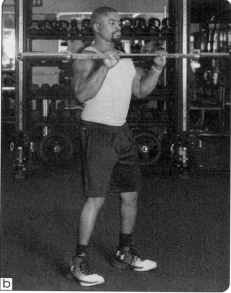

Cable Hammer Curl

As in a hammer grip, your palms face each other as you flex at the elbow during this exercise. This grip allows you to target both the brachialis and brachioradialis musculature.

Equipment

Low-cable rope attachment (alternative: dumbbells or band)

Setup

1. Grip a rope anchored to the bottom of a cable apparatus.
2. Step away from the load until there is tension on your arms at maximal extension (*a*).

Execution

1. Maintain shoulder position and flex at the elbows (*b*).
2. Resist the load as you reverse the direction for the eccentric portion.

Coaching Tips

- This is a rare forearm exercise that allows for the use of the shoulder lock technique, as discussed in chapter 5, Biceps Exercises. Placing your arms against your torso in this way will help to stabilize the shoulder, minimize shoulder muscle fatigue, and allow you to focus on contracting the working arm musculature.
- By your use of a cable attachment, this exercise will offer resistance throughout the full range of motion (ROM). Dumbbells are also effective but may allow you to lose tension at the bottom of the movement (i.e., extreme force delta). Decrease the ROM to maintain tension throughout.
- The dumbbell version of this exercise can be performed seated with back support to minimize the sway of your body.
- Experiment with using palmar and index and thumb grips for maximal muscle targeting.

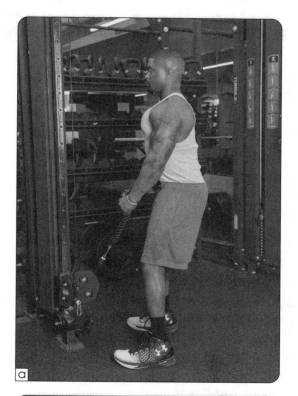

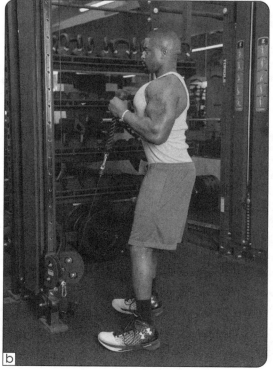

X-Body Hammer Curl

Loaded flexing to see the full depth of your working arm musculature almost makes a mirror required equipment for performing this exercise.

Equipment

Dumbbell (alternative: low-cable rope attachment or band)

Setup

At full elbow extension, pronate the wrist holding the dumbbell, so that your elbow is pointing away from your body (i.e., internal rotation). This is the starting position (*a*).

Execution

1. Flex the elbow to bring the dumbbell across your body so it ends near the center of your chest (*b*).
2. Resist the load to reverse the movement for the eccentric phase.

Coaching Tips

- Instinctively, you may want to use alternating curls, in which you perform a rep with one arm, followed by a rep using the other arm. This makes the exercise easier by allowing the working muscles rest between reps. This is not positive or negative, but rather a variable you should be aware of when trying to optimize stimulation of muscle growth.
- This exercise has the potential for an extreme force delta. You may want to decrease the ROM away from the start of the movement so that the muscle does not lose tension at the bottom.

Variation

This exercise can be performed as a concentration curl. Perform the exercise seated with your elbow resting inside of your knee. This will ensure that tension is maintained throughout the full ROM.

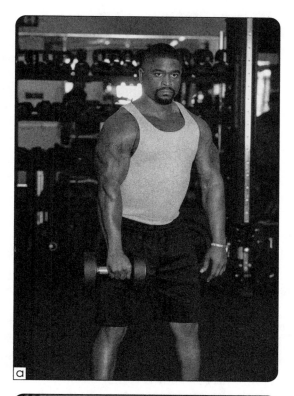

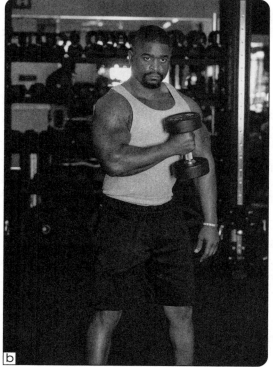

Crush Curl

This single exercise combines two types of equipment to deliver several different contractions. It offers a ton of novel stimuli and will feel "spicy" throughout your arms, shoulders, and chest.

Equipment

- Medicine ball
- Elastic resistance band

Setup

1. Anchor one end of a resistance band at floor level and wrap the other end of the loop around a medicine ball.
2. Grab the sides of the medicine ball with an open hand using a neutral grip so that one side of the band runs across each palm (to ensure that the band doesn't slip off of the medicine ball) (*a*). This is similar to how you would hold a basketball.

Execution

1. Squeeze your hands together as you perform elbow flexion (*b*).
2. The squeeze helps you to maintain stability of the medicine ball and to anchor the band.
3. The cue here is to try to crush the medicine ball as though it were a watermelon (or any fruit that you want to crush, for whatever reason).

Coaching Tips

- Establish your distance from the band anchor point so that there is no slack at the bottom of the exercise and it reaches roughly a 45-degree angle at peak flexion.
- Because of the intense crushing forces, this exercise causes a great pump in your chest and shoulders, as well as your arms.

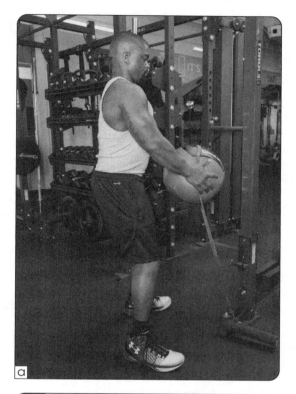

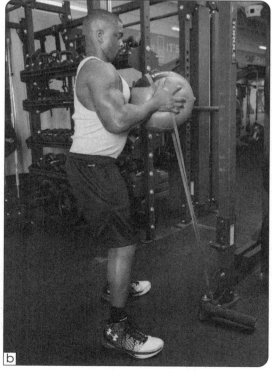

Behind-the-Back Wrist Curl

This is a very small ROM movement that lets you focus on contracting the wrist flexors of the forearm.

Equipment

Barbell

Setup

1. Rack a barbell just below waist height and face away from the bar.
2. Turn your palms toward the bar (i.e., pronate them), back yourself into the bar to grab it, brace your core, and unrack the barbell.
3. The movement begins with your wrist in line with your forearm (i.e., straight) (*a*), from which you perform a concentric wrist flexion.

Execution

1. While maintaining a stable body position, squeeze your forearm flexors to curl the bar (*b*).
2. Reverse direction of the movement for the eccentric portion.

Coaching Tip

Although the ROM is quite small, there are a lot of muscles working during this exercise. Be sure to experiment with the contractions to develop a heightened awareness of these muscles and establish your own strengths, weakness, and preferences. For example, you can try to supinate or pronate (even though your grip is locked) at the top or focus on squeezing more with your pinky or index finger.

Variations

- You can anatomically target the biarticular forearm muscles by using a neutral grip variation of the wrist curl. You will use dumbbells or kettlebells, with your arms hanging straight down at your sides. Rather than walk forward in this traditional dumbbell carry position, simply flex your wrists.
- Let the bar roll down your fingers into a false grip at the end of each rep. In doing so, there should never be a risk of the bar actually slipping out of your hands.

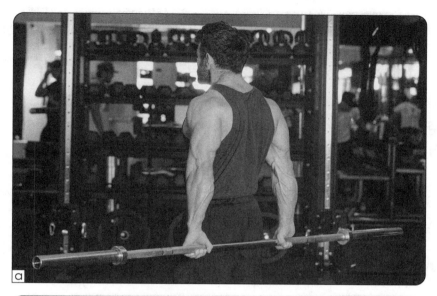

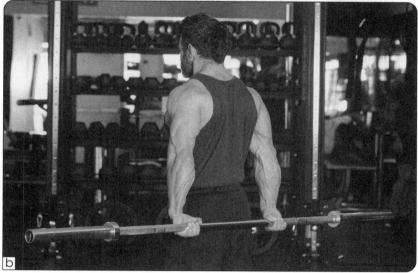

Wenning Wrist Flicks (aka Handshake Curl)

Do not be intimidated by the mighty sound of flicking your wrist. Your forearms are worthy of this isolation exercise.

Equipment

Kettlebell (alternative: dumbbell)

Setup

1. Imagine that you lock the flexed elbow at 90 degrees and perform a handshake motion at the wrist, with an open hand and neutral grip. When you point your fingers up and your thumb toward you, this is known as **radial deviation**. The opposite motion (in which you point your fingers down) is called **ulnar deviation**, and these movements are a great way to think of this next exercise.
2. Sit on a bench with your forearms resting on your thighs so that your wrists are free to move.
3. Grab a kettlebell by the horns with a neutral grip so that it is inverted (*a*). This is the radially deviated starting position from which you begin the eccentric portion of the rep.

Execution

1. Resist the eccentric ulnar deviation so that the bottom of the bell dips downward and faces away from you (*b*).
2. Reverse the direction for the concentric portion of the rep.

Coaching Tip

As you get stronger, you can perform this with one hand gripping the handle of the bell, maintaining a neutral grip.

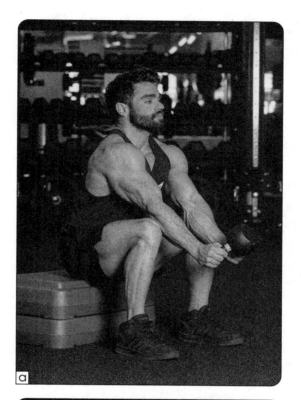

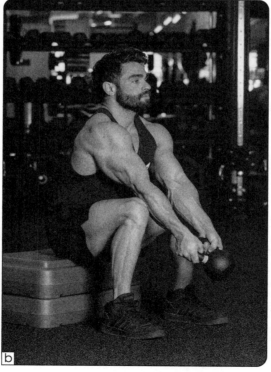

Pronated Dumbbell Curl With Index and Thumb Grip

The execution is nearly identical to the barbell reverse curl, but the unlocked grip provides the additional challenge of having to stabilize your wrist position throughout. In fact, this exercise is excellent for anatomically targeting the pronator muscles of the forearm.

Equipment

Dumbbells

Setup

1. Use a thumb and index grip on the dumbbell, even though you are pronated. This intentionally imbalanced grip results in having more load on the outside (pinky side) of the dumbbell, which forces your pronator muscles to resist supination throughout the movement.
2. Begin with your elbows fully extended (*a*).

Execution

Flex your elbows while maintaining shoulder and wrist position (*b*).

Coaching Tips

- The force potential of elbow flexion is much greater than that of pronation, so your pronation strength and endurance will largely determine the load. This means that you will need to use a relatively light load the first few times you perform this exercise.
- This exercise can be taxing on your grip, so perform it early in your workout before fatigue sets in.

Variations

- Initiate the movement using a neutral grip at the bottom (full elbow extension).
- Pronate as you flex the elbow. This requires active contraction of the pronators, as opposed to an isometric hold.
- Progressively rotate your wrist during the eccentric motion so you end the movement once again with a neutral grip.

Coaching Tips

- This starting wrist position gives the exercise an extreme force delta, with zero force on the muscle in the bottom neutral grip position. You may need to use a slightly frontal shoulder position to ensure that you maintain tension on the arm musculature at the bottom of the exercise.
- Alternatively, you can by avoid full elbow extension, limiting the ROM to that during which you maintain tension.

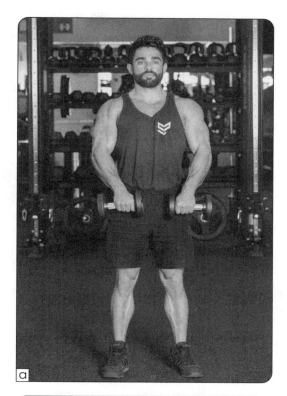

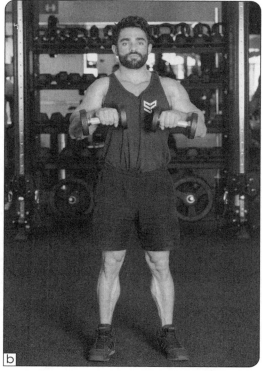

Plate Pinch—Isometric Hold

This simple isometric exercise trains a common type of grip *and* gives you an excuse to make a lot of noise in your gym.

Equipment

Metal training plates

Setup

1. Put two metal plates together so the flat side of each is facing outward.
2. Using one hand, while seated, grip the plates so that they hang straight down beside you, below your thigh. Grip the plates between your flat (extended) fingers and your thumb.
3. These contact points of your hand will each pinch against one plate, and the force of that grip will hold the plates together.
4. As you might expect, this type of grip is known as a **pinch grip**. You can imagine the homologous action of a crab claw or pincer.

Execution

1. While seated with your arm hanging straight down (so that your hands are positioned below the level of your glutes, pinch the plates together.
2. Hold for time.

Coaching Tips

- Perform this exercise last during your workout, because it will absolutely *fry* your grip.
- The seated position decreases the distance that the plates will drop, in the event of a slippage (which happens on occasion). Although the drop is a noisy event, sitting also minimizes the risk of the iron falling onto your foot (or that of others).
- This is a completely isometric movement so you can be creative with your implementation to maintain variety. Along with mixing up the load, using different plates can change the grip width at which you produce the necessary force. For example, holding 30 pounds (13.6 kg) using three 10-pound (4.5 kg) plates feels a lot harder than holding 25- and 5-pound (11.3 and 2.3 kg) plates together.

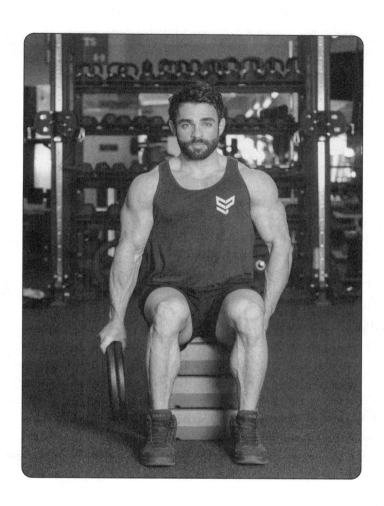

Banded Carries and Variations

If you're looking for a different type of grip killer, adding bands to your carries might be just what you're looking for.

Equipment

- Elastic resistance band or towel
- Plate or kettlebell

Setup

1. Loop a band through a plate or handle of a kettlebell.
2. Place each of the loops over the palm of your hand and wrap your fingers (i.e., hold the band in a crush grip).
3. Stand with your arms hanging at your sides and the band-supported load below your hands (*a*).

Execution

Maintain a fully erect spine and walk slowly with the load.

Coaching Tips

- The bouncing caused by band and the hanging load will create a heightened need for stability for your grip and throughout your entire body.
- You will need to walk slowly.
- You will need to walk smoothly. If you don't know what this means, you *will* when you perform this exercise.

Variations

- A pinky grip can be used to hold the band, which will require you to maintain ulnar deviation throughout the movement. This provides a very intense isometric forearm contraction and may necessitate using a lighter load at first.
- A towel can be used to support the load instead of a band. Although it does not produce as much instability, you are exclusively using a palmar crush grip to hold the load. This means that you don't have the support of your hand anatomy, on which the towel could rest (as it does when using a band).
- If the load is closest to the thumb side, you can experiment with maintaining ulnar deviation or keeping your wrists straight during the carry. The latter will cause the towel to transmit the force of the load over your index finger. This adds a variation to your grip challenge and causes you to isometrically resist ulnar deviation throughout.
- If the load is closest to your pinky finger, you may be most comfortable performing the carry with neutral wrists (*b*). You can experiment with ulnar or radial deviation provided that it does not cause wrist discomfort.

- Instinctively, you may want to try the towel variations using a resistance band. This is not recommended because only the friction of your grip holds the load, and sweat can make the rubber of the band very slippery. If the load slips, it's headed straight toward your foot.

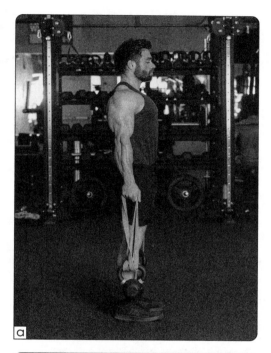

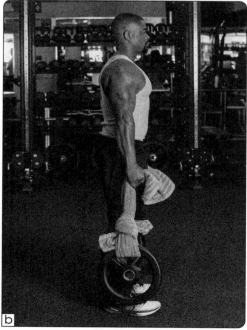

WRAP-UP

We've taken lessons from Matt Wenning and Bruce Lee to find some of the biggest bangs for your buck—anatomically targeted forearm exercises. Although these muscles don't get the love and attention that the biceps and triceps earn, there are few other muscles capable of creating such an immediate impression. Along with building the in-your-face visibility of your forearms, generating a stronger grip with these exercises will help you not only with the rest of your training, but also in everyday life.

Nontraditional Exercises

It may be difficult to imagine a time before hip thrusters and glute bridges were commonly seen in gyms around the world. But it wasn't too long ago, before Dr. Bret Contreras popularized these movements, that they were considered to be nontraditional. In fact, they were often seen as throwbacks to 1980s aerobics studios and toning for tight tushies. The overt sexual nature of these movements generated more than a couple of giggles directed toward the early adopters who performed them. But as you know, that perception has completely changed. This same evolutionary thought process, from rejection to acceptance, also happened for the reintroduction of kettlebells (to North America), calisthenics, and breathing exercises. Now these and countless others are commonplace.

It's important to keep this evolution in mind when learning about and subsequently applying nontraditional techniques. You may get a strange look from someone at the gym when you use them, but this is typically not of concern to early adopters like yourself. You know that the focus is on muscle stimulation and finding the best methods to do so, even if they are a few years ahead of achieving traditional status.

The following exercises began with the end goal of optimizing muscle growth and strength. As a result of this reverse engineering, they go beyond the traditional: concentric and eccentric movements, sets and reps, performed against a gravity resistance. These exercises will help your brain and muscles work together in news ways, which you will experience as rapid gains. They will also refresh your understanding of basic concepts, like contraction, resistance, and strength. Although it may sound daunting, the very best part of this application is that you're going to have fun while doing it. Let's go!

ACCOMMODATING RESISTANCE USING BANDS AND CHAINS

An effective and increasingly popular training technique employs a concept known as **accommodating resistance**. This term applies when the force of the resistance changes throughout the exercise, as a result of your action against it. The best examples of this include elastic resistance and chains, through which the load progressively increases through the concentric range of motion.* Because the tension changes as a result of distance, these techniques are known as **spatially accommodating resistance**. We've seen a few examples of exercises with bands, but really they can be used as a variant with any barbell movement. Classic examples include the bench press and standing biceps curl. Adding chains to the bar is similar, although they will always remain vertical.

Chains hang from the bar (often attached to a smaller chain looped over the bar), starting with most of the links lying on the ground. As you lift the bar, more links come off the ground, progressively adding to your concentric load.

Accommodating Resistance—Applied Intent

Just one more way in which you can benefit from key 5 (targeted focus) happens when you try to contract your muscle rapidly during a rep, in order to activate as many fibers as possible. The idea was reinforced by landmark research from Behm and Sale (1993), who showed that gains were contingent on intent to contract, irrespective of actual movement. This means that you want to try to move quickly, no matter what's happening with the actual movement.

This is where accommodating resistance comes into play, because we are unable to apply this intent with gravity-based implements. If we were to try, the rapid acceleration of the load would cause momentum to quickly take over and you'd have to focus more on *stopping* the load. The good news is that you can take full advantage of this muscle activation technique through the use of the various accommodating resistance techniques shown in this chapter. For example, you will reap the greatest benefit when you try to accelerate concentrically during a banded biceps curl or against isokinetic eccentric resistance.

We focus on anchoring bands from below, but they can also be hung from above to provide a deload at the bottom of the range of motion (ROM), as exemplified by arm-focused pull-ups in chapter 10. Either way, the same principle applies: progressively increasing resistance throughout the concentric ROM.

Another benefit of accommodating resistance is that it allows you to change the strength curve of an exercise, so you're challenged at different parts of the movement. An ideal example would be to change an exercise that normally has an extreme force delta so that you'd be able to maintain tension throughout the full range of motion (ROM). If you were to perform preacher curls with a band anchored in front of you, the result would be that you would have tension at the top of the movement (when the band is maximally stretched). Lastly, they can just be a great psychological change from traditional training.

Things to Remember

- Bands wear out and eventually break. Be sure to inspect them for wear before every use.
- When anchoring bands, ensure that the anchor point is stable. Do not have another human hold the band to anchor it (for me and a colleague, this point was emphasized when the colleague found himself with a broken nose by as a result of doing so).
- Chains are a pain to haul around between workouts because they can be very heavy (which really is the point). They are also very noisy, which is why some gyms do not allow their use.
- Chains will naturally oscillate as you perform the lift, which can be an interesting novel stimulus if it is managed. You can minimize unwanted movement by ensuring that some length of chain remains on the ground throughout the entire lift, which adds a little stability.

Banded Preacher Curl

There are few exercises that benefit you more from the addition of elastic accommodating resistance. Because this exercise has an extreme force delta, typically resulting in a rest period at maximal flexion, the band helps to reveal any weaknesses you've induced created by this instinct. The magnitude of the stress stimulus and resulting growth makes it worth the pain of the setup and execution.

Equipment

Barbell and band(s)

Setup

1. Loop one or two bands around or through a stable low anchor point, so that they will stretch maximally at your maximal elbow flexion.
2. Loop the ends of the bands symmetrically onto the bar to provide balanced resistance.
3. Grip the bar and sit back so that your arms are fully in contact with the pad (*a*). Note that this does not mean that you should sit down on a seat.

Execution

1. Flex the elbow to curl the weight (*b*).
2. Maintain shoulder and arm position throughout.

Coaching Tips

- If it is not possible to perform the movement without developing slack in the bands at maximal extension (i.e., the bottom of the movement), simply end the ROM just prior to this point.
- Focus your intent on contracting the muscle quickly. Although you might perform the concentric movement faster than normal on the first few reps, the bands will eliminate the momentum at the top of the movement.
- The bands not only increase tension throughout the movement, but they might increase time under tension if you've been resting at the top. This will create a surprising degree of fatigue and subsequent stimulus, so be sure to start with the lightest bands and reduce your standard training weight.
- If you're experienced with standard preacher curls, the addition of the bands will completely change the feel of the exercise. This is especially true if you perform the traditional preacher rest at the top of the movement. The bands not only eliminate the undesirable rest, but they create *maximal* tension at this point.

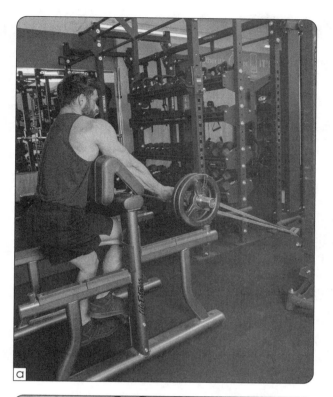

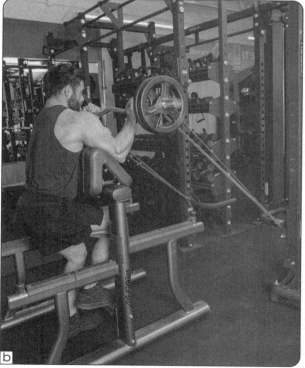

Banded Triceps Push-Down

Spatially accommodating resistance can be used with other types of resistance or on its own. A one-arm push-down is a great example of how solo band work can provide unique advantages for your growth.

Equipment

Band

Setup

1. Loop one end of a band around a stable, high-anchor point.
2. Face the band.
3. Using a neutral grip, place your hand inside the bottom of the hanging loop, using a pinky grip to transmit force during execution. Wrap your fingers around the palm side of the band for stability (*a*). Your arm should be roughly vertical with your elbow at your side.

Execution

Maintain shoulder position and quickly extend your elbow by flexing your triceps.

Coaching Tips

- Using a neutral pinky grip is helpful to support the resistance across the wrist. Other grips can be used but will require greater wrist stability.
- For eccentric overload, the nonworking arm can help to achieve maximal extension (*b*), after which the working arm performs the eccentric movement alone.
- The eccentric overload can be exaggerated further by stretching the band while maintaining the fully extended position with the nonworking hand. For example, with your elbow extended you could step backward away from the anchor point, bend at the waist, or partially squat. Once the band is stretched to the desired length, the working arm performs the eccentric movement alone. Return to the starting standing position, with minimal tension on the band for another rep.

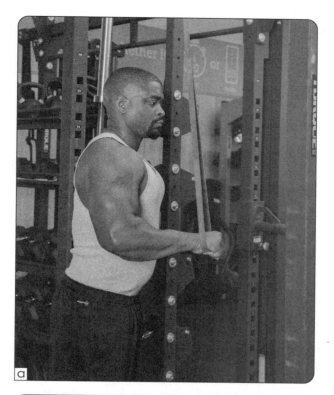

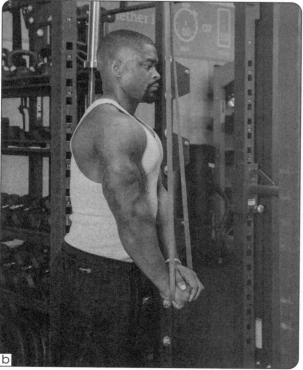

ACCOMMODATING RESISTANCE USING THE TREADMILL

In previous chapters we discussed the **eccentric paradox**, which reflects the fact that we're stronger eccentrically but almost always exert less force during this phase. This means that we're leaving a lot of natural strength and growth stimulus on the table every time we perform a rep. In an attempt to tap into this growth potential, computer-controlled machines have been developed to move the bar at a predetermined speed, no matter how hard you push. Imagine a seated bench press that performs the exercise by itself! Your goal would be to sit on the machine as normal and push against the moving handles.

These machines are called **isokinetic equipment** (*iso* = same, *kinetic* = movement) and have been used in the physical therapy setting for decades. Although they solve the eccentric paradox, they are prohibitively expensive, which forces us to put our innovation hat on and find our own isokinetic workaround.

The solution is to use a computer-controlled isokinetic device found in almost every commercial gym: the treadmill.

To apply key 5 with the eccentric exercises described in this chapter, remember your goal is not to simply resist the movement of the belt but instead to attempt to perform a concentric movement even though your arm is being forced in the opposite direction by the movement of the treadmill belt. This known as a **forced eccentric movement**, or overwhelming eccentric movement, and it's going to be a strange feeling at first. Applying this concept not only helps us to think differently about resistance, but the exercises serve as powerful, untapped stimuli for adaptation.

Application Essentials

There are four reasons why you'll love this type of resistance. The first two results are physical in nature (microtargeted growth and fast gains), but the others can be described as experiential and mind blowing (rewiring your brain and a paradigm shift).

Microtargeted Growth

The eccentric portion of a rep is where much of the growth-stimulating micro damage happens to muscle, during each exercise. This has been limited by your concentric movements and gravity-based loads, but forced eccentric movements allow you to tap into your organic eccentric strength for a more powerful growth stimulus.

Fast Gains

Strength increases with forced eccentric training happen faster than you might expect. This is similar to the way in which concentric strength gains often come very quickly when someone first begins strength training. Rapid adaptation happens because your brain and nervous system are learning how to better communicate with your muscles. Although you've probably been through this with traditional concentric-constrained training, that type of neural strength adaptation still hasn't happened with eccentric contractions. As a result, you will quickly become stronger, and these reps will be more comfortable and come to feel more locked in. This means that even if you have decades of training experience, you'll quickly get stronger as your body adapts to this brand-new stimulus.

Rewiring Your Brain

Right now our brain and muscles really only understand gravity-based resistance, so the idea of a different type of resistance would mean swapping a dumbbell for a kettlebell (both of which are nearly identical gravity-based loads). In contrast, applying isokinetic and forced eccentric exercises helps to expand the breadth of our ability to produce force against different types of resistance—which you may not have known to exist, until now! This breadth extends to the fact that these exercises apply forces that adapt to you throughout the rep. These action–reaction forces (which you may remember hearing about in physics class) put them in another subgroup of accommodating resistance, called **force-accommodating** (also known as [aka] tonically accommodating). This means that the force of the resistance (exerted against you) changes based on the amount of force you're exerting. These changes happen instantly, in real time, during every rep. Training doesn't get any more personalized than this.

Paradigm Shift

The use of isokinetic and force-accommodating resistance via a treadmill induces a fundamental paradigm shift for the way in which we perceive the stimulation adaptation of muscle and applied resistance. Stated differently, it helps us to think differently about how to get bigger gains. Sure, we'll always need to perform consecutive reps of concentric-constrained gravity-based loads, but we don't need to limit ourselves to this anymore. We may

SideBarr

Force-accommodating resistance also happens every time you sit down and with every step you take. The more force you exert, the harder the ground pushes back.

not have known that these limits existed, but just reading about this type of novel application shatters the barriers that have been imposed by our primitive Iron Age tradition. The destination? Optimized and personalized adaptation—whether it's getting bigger, faster, stronger, or leaner; or going longer. This shift in thinking all comes down to *how you can achieve the best results for you.*

Summary of Benefits

1. Microtargeted growth
2. Rapid strength increases
3. Increased breadth of force production
4. Advanced awareness of how to produce force and stimulate muscle

Advanced Accommodating Application

Isokinetic resistance training can be used to optimize yet another type of accommodating resistance, which is called **kinetically accommodating resistance**. This means that your ability to exert force (aka strength, aka **force potential**) changes as a result of the speed of contraction. The faster you are forced eccentrically, the more force you can produce. In fact, fast eccentrics offer your greatest ability to produce force and subsequent stimulus for growth. Unfortunately, once again, gravity prevents us from ever taking advantage of this, because the only to move faster during the negative portion of a lift is to exert *less* force.

For example, imagine that you're performing a barbell bench press and want to perform a fast negative. After reaching full lockout, how do you get the bar down quickly? You have to exert minimal eccentric force, essentially letting the bar drop. Although many people train this way naturally, hoping that the recoil of their rib cage will give them a boost on the next concentric, this common cheat does not tap into your maximal force potential. To actually take advantage of your maximal strength (i.e., fast eccentric strength), you have to use kinetically accommodating resistance (i.e., isokinetic resistance). *This is the greatest amount of force that human beings can generate, although few people actually do so. You have this maximal strength potential right now. You simply need the right type of resistance to tap into it.*

It is unlikely that you've ever experienced the magnitude of force output that you're capable of achieving with slow eccentric overload, but fast eccentric movements increase this force output to an even greater extent. For this reason, applying the speed component to eccentric training is an advanced training stimulus that should be applied only after developing mastery over slow forced eccentrics. When you can consistently attempt to contract concentrically during an eccentric overload, the kinetic variable be introduced. A common error, called **premature acceleration**, happens when you introduce speed too soon. The result is that you'll never learn how to contract maximally against an overwhelming force, and you'll miss out on the growth potential. Remember that when it comes to forced eccentrics, *practice makes powerful!*

Types of Accommodation

1. *Accommodating resistance.* A resistance that changes based on external factors.
2. *Spatially accommodating.* Change with distance of movement (e.g., elastic bands and chains).
3. *Force accommodating.* Change with the amount of force you apply (e.g., isokinetic resistance).
4. *Kinetically accommodating.* Change with speed and your subsequent force application (e.g., isokinetic resistance).

Treadmill Press

The movement of the treadmill press is similar to the eccentric portion of a one-arm dumbbell press, using the isokinetic movement of the treadmill belt as resistance.

Setup

1. While standing on the treadmill, set it to one mile per hour (1.6 km/hr) or slower and carefully step off without changing direction (as though you were running on the belt), and set up in quadruped stance (i.e., on your hands and knees). Place the hand of your working arm on the moving belt toward the head end of the treadmill (where the control panel is) (*a*).

2. Your other hand can serve as support on the side of the treadmill, safely away from the moving belt.

Execution

1. Begin with your shoulder flexed and your elbow at maximal extension (i.e., the top of the ROM), just as in the top of a shoulder press.

2. As you push the palm of your open hand into the belt, try to concentrically flex the shoulder and extend the elbow (*b*).

3. Your hand and arm will be forced backward, replicating an eccentric portion of a one-arm shoulder press.

4. When the desired ROM is complete, simply lift your hand from the belt.

5. Rest as long as necessary to perform the next rep with full focus, and then repeat.

Coaching Tips

- As you perform forced eccentric reps, your nervous system will quickly fall back into the habit of passively resisting the movement, as opposed to trying to move concentrically. This habit has likely been ingrained in you after thousands of reps, so don't worry about it; it's just going to happen. What's important is that you become aware of it and adapt your behavior. When you regain awareness that you're being passive, switch your focus back to the *intent* of actively performing a concentric movement, and you'll immediately feel the difference.

- Use a spotter who can stop the belt if necessary.

- Nothing other than your flat palm should even come close to the belt. All jewelry should be removed, and loose clothing should be tucked or removed.

- Start to incorporate these exercises with a very slow movement on the belt. If your full ROM rep duration is less than one second, the belt is moving too quickly. To get the feel of contraction and to rewire your nervous system, the belt needs to be moving slowly for the first several weeks.

- To decrease the risk of excessive soreness, use a partial ROM starting with the shortest muscle length (this is always the default starting position and is described for each exercise). As you become more experienced you can increase to ROM.

- One downside of this type of training is that it lacks an objective measure of resistance and subsequent progress. This is why it becomes especially important for you to understand that as your strength progressively increases each week, and you apply this strength during each rep, the resistance applied by the belt will also increase. So as long as you're putting in the effort, your strength will continually grow, even if you can't directly observe it via a numerical value (e.g., throwing another plate onto the bar). The good news is that you *will* be able to see the resulting hypertrophy and strength gains across other exercises.

- Avoid the temptation to use progressive weekly increases in treadmill speed as a desperate surrogate for numerical improvement. This premature acceleration happens because we've been conditioned to associate the feeling of progression with the act of increasing a number on a machine (or on a barbell, etc.). Break this conditioning by maintaining focus on stimulating your muscle on every rep. This allows you to rely on your own effort for weekly progression, which personalizes your training even further.

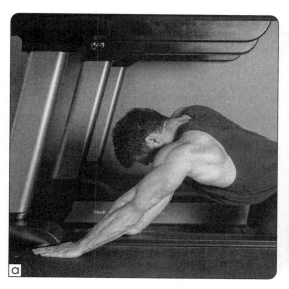
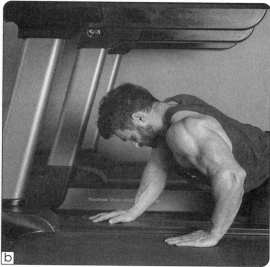

Treadmill Row

This exercise uses the opposite movement of the triceps press, so you set up in quadruped stance beside the treadmill facing toward the back end.

Setup

1. Begin with your elbow flexed and arm at your side, as though you have just completed the concentric phase of a cable pull-down.
2. Your support hand will brace on the side of the treadmill, safely away from the moving belt (*a*).

Execution

1. Create isometric tension in your arm and back and press your hand into the moving belt.
2. Attempt to actively contract concentrically as your arm is pulled eccentrically (*b*).

Coaching Tip

Among the elements that make this exercise unique is the fact that you are pushing your hand into the belt while trying to "row" (adduct) your elbow to your side. This is employed as a back exercise, but you're also going to feel it in your triceps. Recall that the long head of the triceps crosses the shoulder, and its actions include elbow extension and shoulder extension. Because the opposite of both of these actions is imposed by the treadmill row, the movement acts as a double eccentric movement, which activates the long head in a way that no other exercise can.

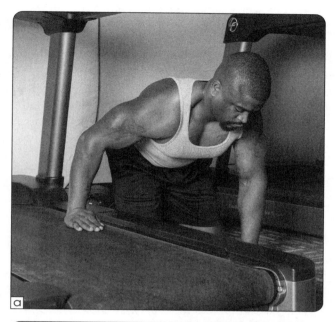

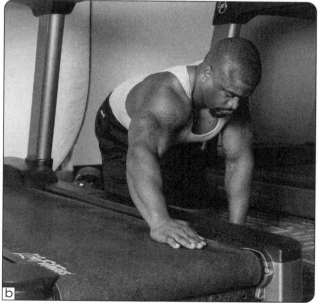

Barr Fly

In chapter 3, we dissected the traditional dumbbell pec fly and uncovered its many weaknesses. Because the shoulder adduction movement is fundamental to chest development and *should* be a good fit with anatomically targeted training, I've been eager to find an alternative. By sheer coincidence, performing the movement with isokinetic treadmill resistance seems to solve *every* problem created by the old exercise. Moreover, the newer version seems to go further, by optimizing the movement in every category (see table 7.1).

Collectively, the take-home message isn't to vilify DB flys or shamelessly promote Barr flys. The key here lies in the difference between simply following Iron Age tradition, versus optimization through analysis, insight, and innovation.

Table 7.1 Comparing Dumbbell Pectoralis Flys and Barr Flys

		DB fly	Barr fly
	ROM	Limited	Full
	Force delta	Extreme	Optimal
Stimuli	ROM of load stimulus	50%	Optimal
	Force accommodating	Paradoxical	Optimal
	Kinetically accommodating	Paradoxical	Optimal
		DB fly	**Barr fly**
	Scapular mobility	Pinned	Free
Safety	Joint-vulnerable loading	Maximal	Organic
	Muscle-vulnerable loading	Maximal	Organic
	Momentum at vulnerable ROM	Yes	None

SideBarr

I'm not sure which of the following I like best about the name *Barr fly*:

1. The intentionally absurd eponymous nature;
2. The homonym that conjures images of Cliff and Norm from the 1980s TV show *Cheers;*
3. That the exercise is somewhat antithetical to barbell training, despite the implication that it uses a bar; or
4. The fact that when you say it quickly it sounds like "barf lies."

Setup

1. Stand beside the treadmill facing the belt and assume a quadruped position.
2. Use your non working arm to support your body weight on the side of the treadmill.
3. If you are using your left arm as the working limb (for example), the belt should be moving from right to left in front of you.
4. With your torso nearly parallel to the belt, adduct your shoulder to bring your arm across the body, while maintaining a stable shoulder position. If you were to look down at your arm in this position, you will likely see it form approximately a 45-degree angle with your chest. Although you might achieve greater adduction by popping your shoulder forward, this would be an unstable and potentially unsafe position. Allow your stable shoulder position to naturally dictate the starting position of the exercise.

Execution

1. With your elbow fully extended and shoulder adducted, press your hand into the center of the belt (*a*).
2. Attempt to actively adduct the arm, as the belt forces you eccentrically into abduction (*b*).

Coaching Tips

- Maintain an extended elbow throughout.
- Although you might not actually feel it, be aware that you're producing a huge amount of force during this movement.
- This requires a surprising amount of core strength to maintain stability and resist rotation. Even though it is isometric for these muscles, you'll probably feel your core the next day.

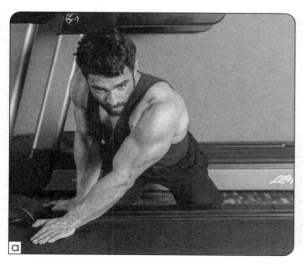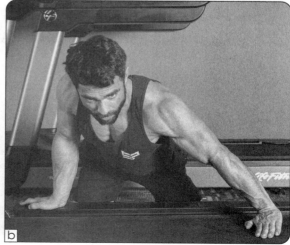

Flexy Training

One of the best ways to ensure maximal long-term arm development is through strengthening your shoulder stabilizers. Using bands to support a hanging load, or bars that are designed to flex and bend, such as a bamboo bar, are fun ways to accomplish this while exposing your muscles to a new, contractile stimulus.

Equipment

Barbell, bands, and weight plates (alternative: bamboo bar)

Setup

1. Loop one band through a light plate and repeat with a second band and second plate.
2. Secure the bands to opposite ends of the bar so that the load is balanced (one plate per side).

Execution

As the bar moves throughout any exercise the plates will shift and bounce while hanging in the bands, the force of which is amplified by the bar.

Coaching Tips

- For the sake of novelty you can experiment with this strategy on any barbell exercise, including isolated biceps and triceps movements.
- For its intended purpose of developing shoulder stability and for long-term physique development, it's best to start with a compound exercise like the bench press.

Variation

Performing the bench press with a flexy bar is just as described with a standard bar in chapter 4, ensuring that you have a spotter. This is a perfect opportunity to use the checklist and practice your technique. The load should feel very light, because you're stimulating the shoulder stabilizers—*not* trying to fatigue your triceps or pectoralis muscles (see the image on the next page).

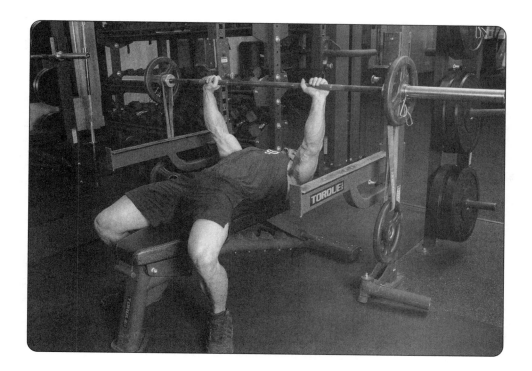

Panda Training

Because we use light weight for this movement, it can be hard to know when to terminate the set. You may only come to notice creeping fatigue when it begins to induce a strange horizontal oscillation of the bamboo bar. When this fatigue happens, the bar will shift back and forth, toward your head, then toward your waist, and then back toward the head. This is caused by the progressive fatigue of the shoulder stabilizers allowing the flex of the bar and elastic force of the bands to take over (this devolution morphs the exercise into **panda training**). The amplitude of this oscillation increases with each fatigued rep, which can result in your losing control of the bar (aka dumping). If you dump toward your face, you're eating bamboo. If you dump toward your waist, you can't reproduce. Don't be a panda!

SLED TRAINING

This implement can be any load that provides resistance while you pull or push it across the ground. One application is to perform prolonged physical activity against a heavy resistance for cardio or general physical preparation. Alternatively, sleds are used for recovery work because of the concentric-only nature of their movement (see figure 7.1). We'll discuss this specific application in a little more detail with three-phase feeder workouts in chapter 8, Recovery.

When used for recovery workouts, sled movements are optimized by using longer duration contractions and low concentric tension. One goal is to locally increase blood flow to the working muscle without inducing further mechanical stress. For this reason, sleds are a natural fit because the damage-inducing eccentric portion of the movement is eliminated. Also, contractions performed with a one- to two-second concentric movement and a one- to two-second isometric hold at the peak offer a consistent, prolonged tension and brief occlusion of blood flow that will subsequently increase nutrient delivery. This point was really hammered home for me when discussing sled work with elite powerlifter and performance coach, Tasha "Wolf" Whelan, who said "Isometrics are a hugely underutilized component of arm training. They are great for increasing metabolic demand and can help to facilitate recovery adaptation" (Tasha Whelan, pers. comm.).

Some people have described the desired contractions to be performed with sled-based movements as fast, as though you are trying to accelerate the sled (aka grip and rip). Although it is not generally incorrect, this suggestion directly contradicts our specific goals of recovery adaptation for two reasons.

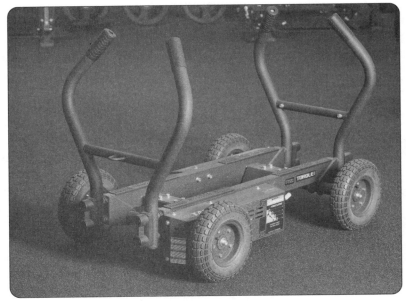

Figure 7.1   A sled with wheels.

1. It places a huge amount of tension on the working muscle at the most stretched position, which is where it is most susceptible to muscle damage. This damage is part of the stress we want during normal training but not during a recovery session.

2. Secondly, the momentum results in the near elimination of tension throughout the rest of the ROM. If you're trying to get a pump, brief tension isn't the best tool for the job.

When choosing your exercises, consider performing similar movements to those that you executed during your last lift. This will help to mimic the muscle fiber recruitment and facilitate their recovery adaptation.

Attach a long connector such as a suspension trainer to a weighted sled and grab the handles of the connector. With tension on the connector, anchor your lower body and perform the upper body movement against the resistance of the sled, which will be dragged toward you. For the next rep, you walk away from the sled to reestablish tension and repeat.

Chest Press

The chest press is one of the most common movements performed during sled work.

Setup

Face away from the sled, use a staggered stance for stability (*a*).

Execution

Perform a triceps-focused press (*b*).

Coaching Tip

The additional pump in your shoulders and chest can be seen as a bonus.

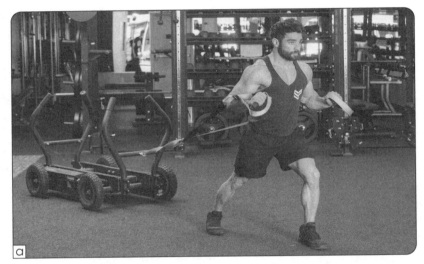

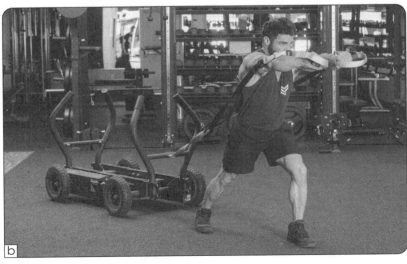

Lock and Walk

If you have a relatively weak lockout or performed end-ROM work during your last session, you can use the lock and walk technique.

Setup

Face away from the sled and perform a chest press to take any slack out of the connector (*a*).

Execution

Walk forward with the sled behind you and maintain the lockout position (*b*).

Coaching Tip

The goal is to maintain steady tension on your extended triceps by walking at a consistent pace.

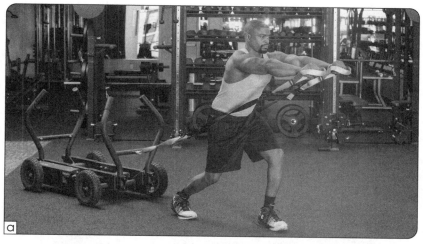

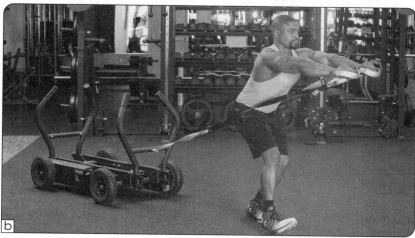

Triceps Extension Variations

These movements can be performed with either anterior or neutral shoulder position variations, which changes with the setup phase based on position. The execution phase is the same for both.

Anterior Shoulder Position

Setup

Face away from the sled with your elbows flexed and your shoulders flexed so that your elbows are slightly higher than your shoulders (i.e., arms above parallel to the ground) (*a*).

Execution

Extend the elbows by squeezing the triceps against the resistance of the sled (*b*).

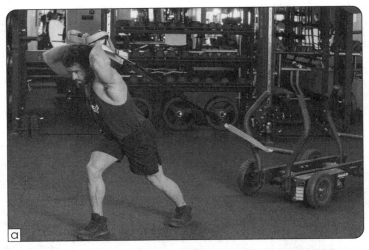

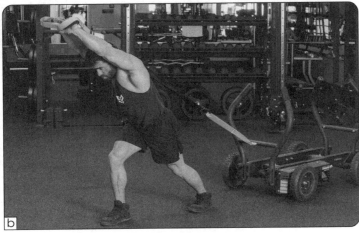

Neutral Shoulder Position

Setup

1. Face the sled and push your hips back to bend at the waist so that your chest is facing the ground.
2. Grip the connector handles with your arms at your sides and elbows fully flexed (*c*).

Execution

Extend the elbows by squeezing the triceps against the resistance of the sled (*d*).

Coaching Tip

Some shoulder movement is inevitable.

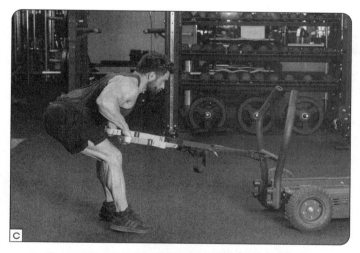

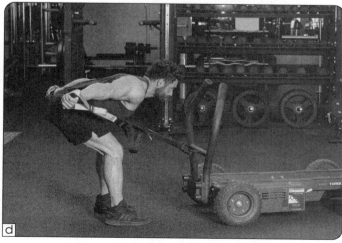

Sled Curl Variations

Biceps movements involve relatively short ROM but can be performed with any of the three shoulder positions.

Frontal Position

Setup

For the frontal shoulder position, face the sled and hold the connector with your arms roughly parallel to the ground (*a*).

Execution

Maintain the starting shoulder position and flex your elbows to pull the sled toward you (*b*).

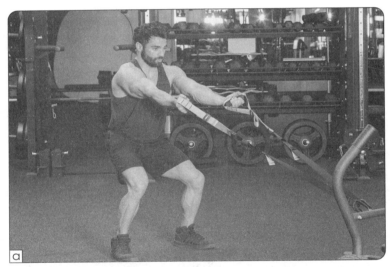

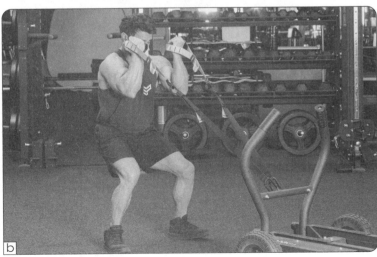

Neutral and Posterior Positions

Setup

1. For the neutral and posterior shoulder positions, face away from the sled and hold the connector at or slightly behind your hips (*a*).
2. Use a staggered stance for stability.

Execution

Flex your elbows by squeezing your arm musculature (*b*).

Coaching Tip

For the neutral shoulder position, you may be able to use the shoulder lock technique, which can help mitigate shoulder fatigue.

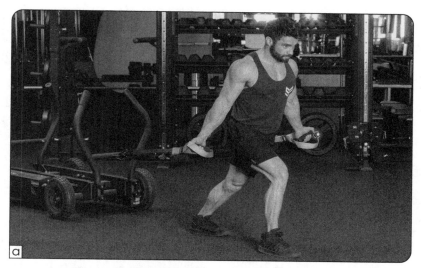

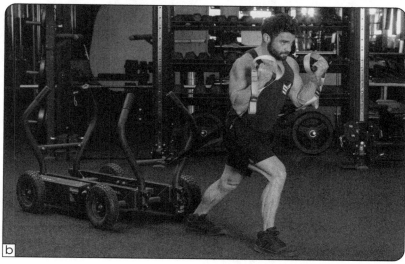

TRADITIONAL EXERCISES PERFORMED NONTRADITIONALLY

Rope Climb and Sled Variation

Like a pommel horse, high suspended ropes were an old-school physical culture implement that used to be standard issue in gyms everywhere. If your facility doesn't have a rope attached to the ceiling, you may have access to a machine designed to let you replicate rope climbing. Although the exercise starts off concentrically only, it could become eccentric-only on the descent, if you allow it. For this to occur, rather than using your legs to assist on the way down, slowly lower yourself by squeezing as much of your arm musculature as you can.

The ascent of traditional rope climbs can also have its difficulty increased by using your arms only to climb, while bringing your knees up to hip level and holding throughout.

This arm-centric movement can be replicated using a sled, which allows you greater concentric control over the load and subsequent difficulty. Face the sled, bend (i.e., push your hips back so your chest faces the ground), and use the connector as a rope (*a*) that you pull hand over hand, just as you would in a climb. The connector will likely be short enough that you'll have to step back after a pull from each hand (*b*).

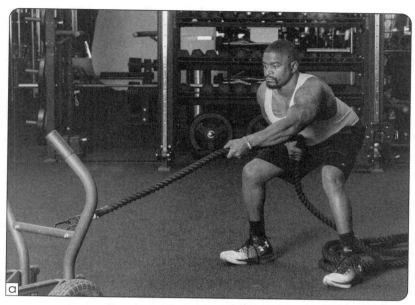

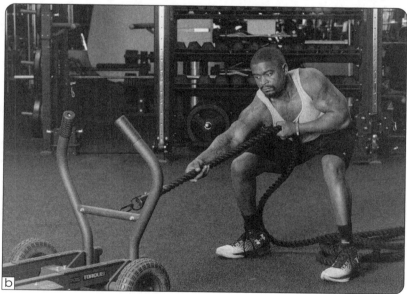

Overhead Triceps Walk

Equipment

- High suspended rope or barbell
- Squat rack

Setup

1. This movement involves progressively walking your body downward along the length of a rope or slanted barbell, hand over hand (as though you are shimmying along a pipe), while also performing small elbow flexion and extension movements. The starting position is similar to that of an overhead triceps extension, but rather than a cable attachment, you're gripping a static overhead rope or barbell.

2. The rope setup requires only an overhead attachment (a), but the more complicated barbell setup warrants greater detail. Place one safety bar in the rack just below chest height and the other at roughly the height of your lower abs. Place the barbell in the rack on the uneven safety bars, so that it is angled downward. The barbell should be secured by the notch created from the inside of its bushing (aka the knobby thing) and terminus of the grip area on the higher safety bar (b). Stand inside the rack facing toward the lower end of the barbell and ensure that it is secure.

3. Push your hips back to bend at the waist so that your torso is nearly parallel to the ground directly under the barbell. Grip the now overhead barbell with a neutral grip. You'll want your hands touching each other, so that the pinky side of your closest hand is up against the index finger and thumb of your farther hand. Some of your weight will now be supported by the barbell overhead, and your arms should be covering your ears.

Execution

1. The movement begins by "walking" one hand down the implement away from you so that it grips the implement just on the other side of your other hand.

2. As each hand alternately travels down the implement, perform a slight elbow flexion and extension by rocking your body forward and backward, respectively.

Coaching Tips

- You can set the safety bars at any height difference, although starting with a smaller difference is preferred to make this challenging exercise more manageable.

- The rope offers a greater challenge because of its mobility. The more vertical your starting body position, the easier the exercise will be.
- You can walk as far down the bar (or rope) as you prefer, and back up if you'd like. As with every eccentric-heavy exercise, it is recommended that you start with low volume and adjust based on the extent of the resulting delayed-onset muscle soreness.

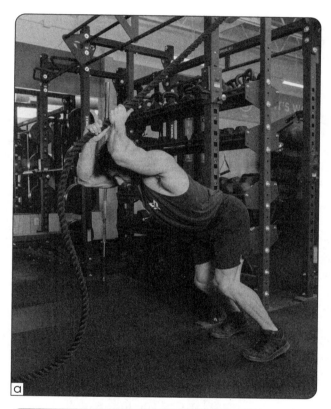

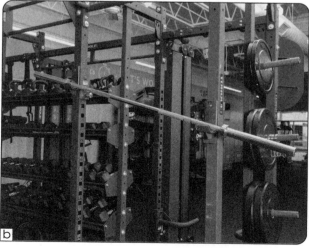

Rice Bucket Challenge

A staple of grapplers and climbers around the world, manipulating your hands in a bucket of uncooked rice can be a fun way to improve your forearms' size and your grip strength. Fill any bucket with rice. Larger buckets (e.g., five-gallon) will allow you to use both arms at once if you prefer. The working hand should dive into the rice with fingers extended. Once buried, you can perform concentric movements of the hand, wrist, and shoulder against the resistance of the rice. An example is to perform a crush by gripping the rice as you would a bar, followed by opening your hand and spreading your fingers. Note that because this is concentric only, you may feel a burn from the working muscles but are unlikely to incur delayed-onset muscle soreness.

Coaching Tips

- The deeper your hands are buried, the greater the resistance.
- Sand can be used as an alternative to rice but is more likely to cause a muddy mess as you perspire.
- Dry your hands and arms before plunging them into the rice to minimize sticking (and the subsequent mess when you remove them).
- Keep a lid on the bucket when not in use to prevent general contamination.
- Have a broom and dustpan nearby. You *will* need them.

WRAP-UP

It's likely that after reading this chapter, your training will never be the same. You've seen how to tap into a level of strength that few humans will ever do. The resulting stimulation of muscle growth and strength gain will reflect that accomplishment. Better yet, you've seen how to expand your breadth of force generation and escape beyond the limits of gravity. Along with this comes a fundamental upgrade of the neural software, advancing your very understanding of resistance training. Collectively, the means to accomplish these feats may seem unusual at first, but by applying them, you'll come to see that you're simply ahead of the crowd.

Recovery Optimization

If you've tried to learn about recovery from fitness-related media, you may have found the information seems limited to only the following tropes: glycogen restoration, hydration, and sleep cycles. These ideas were great, but they predate the existence of texting. As always, we'll fill that information vacuum with meaty goodness that you can apply to your physique right away.

Let's begin the upgrade with a statement that evokes such a strong emotional reaction that I can only refer to it as the shocker. *You don't want recovery.* It's controversial enough that I may find myself the target of nerd rage on social media, but consider the statement in the context of these three common scenarios and their solutions.

1. If you're training to maintain muscle size rather than increase it, then you may be concerned with accelerating recovery. But remember that recovery is merely a return to baseline (but not going beyond), which is not your goal. You want growth. Solution: upgrade your recovery adaptation.

2. If your recovery adaptation is impaired due to excessive training volume or frequency, this will likely manifest as general fatigue or burnout, rather than muscle soreness (for example). These are not muscle-based issues, nor can they be fixed with traditional recovery interventions. Solution: fix your training.

3. If your recovery adaptation is impaired due to basic lifestyle factors, such as chronically inadequate sleep or nutritional deficiencies, your solution lies outside of training. Again, these issues will not be fixed by slapping a commonly touted recovery technique onto your program. Solution: fix your lifestyle.

The exception to these reasons comes with the muscle soreness that accompanies the eccentric overload training (used to optimize structural growth). Although you'll probably come to love a bit of post-eccentric, delayed-onset muscle soreness (DOMS), it should not be excessive or chronic. Although the techniques described in this chapter may help, you'll see how to keep DOMS manageable via personalization in upcoming chapters.

In order to accelerate your arm development, I'll reveal some of my own lab-based research experiences along with how to use the surprising results for improved recovery adaptation. We'll cover easy-to apply interventions to help get you started today and destroy a couple of **zombie myths** (i.e., those that refuse to die, not myths about zombies) along the way.

It's important to remember the Selye recovery adaptation curve (from chapter 2) and the cautionary tale of using blue shifting techniques in an attempt to accelerate recovery. With that in mind, we'll explore interventions that facilitate the body's organic recovery or adaptation response, rather than trying to blunt it. To differentiate them from traditional destructive recovery methods, those presented here are called **adaptive recovery** (aka **progressive recovery**) techniques. So rather than blindly chasing recovery, we'll use what we learned about adaptive targeting (key 3) and precision microtargeting (key 4) in order to maximize your arm development.

SYMPATHETIC SHIFTING

The body has two primary systems to consider for recovery adaptation, and like a physiological sniper, we'll optimize our effectiveness by targeting interventions for each. Muscle is the most obvious target, but we can't neglect the most integrated system of all, the **nervous system** (aka the **central nervous system [CNS]**). You can think of it as the body's internal wiring that causes muscle to contract, but it's even more important than that because it's related to our mood, as well as our levels of energy and stress.

One practical example of this is the preworkout activation phase (from chapter 3) that gets the **sympathetic nervous system** (aka **fight or flight**) going to facilitate an intense workout. If we stay in this mode for too long, which can happen with chronic stress and inadequate recovery, we'll enter a physiological state of **overtraining**. This dreaded state results in a prolonged fatigue and mood disturbance that should be avoided like that guy at your gym who asks for a spot but then makes you do all the work.

So, while sympathetic activation is great for a short period of time, we want to balance that stimulation with a more relaxed alertness by shifting toward the **parasympathetic** (aka **rest and digest**) side of the spectrum after the lift. The problem with this **sympathetic shifting** is that the emotional stresses of everyday life push us into being chronically stimulated, anxious, or just stressed out. When we live on the sympathetic side of the spectrum, we're always in overdrive, and it becomes harder to find anything left to activate for a workout. It also means that we have chronically high levels of the stress hormone cortisol, which can increase muscle breakdown muscle and suppress immune response. The worst-case scenario happens when we exceed our limits for too long, and our engine burns out. This is overtraining, and when it happens it can be hard to get out of bed, let alone get up for a workout.

This is the basis for the popular book *Why Zebras Don't Get Ulcers*. We want to be more like zebras, who remain ulcer free because they don't experience the chronic stresses that we primates do. Further, by maintaining a baseline chill attitude, they are able turn on their CNS (i.e., activate it) immediately when they need to perform (e.g., escape from a hungry lion). If we extrapolate these ideas to ourselves, sympathetic shifting could lead to more effective workouts, but more importantly a happier, healthier life.

THE NASA RECOVERY PLAN

The first clues for this recovery technique came from my National Aeronautics and Space Administration research experience at the Johnson Space Center, which investigated the connections between muscle and the nervous system. For our purposes, it pertained to the use of sensory input in an attempt to decrease muscle loss, which is critical for long-duration spaceflight (i.e., going to Mars and beyond).

It turns out that something as simple as touch provides enough sensory input to the nervous system that it affects other tissues, like muscle. In our case, chronic touch of the foot provided enough stimulation that muscle mass was maintained, even during simulated microgravity. This means that even though the muscle itself had no direct stimulation (which would normally cause it to shrivel like a punctured balloon), the nervous system was able to step in and disrupt the accelerated muscle breakdown.

We can use this idea by removing sensory input for brief periods of time after a workout to decrease the load on the nervous system and restore a calm alert state. When you combine this with controlled diaphragmatic breathing (aka belly breathing), your body shifts from a sympathetic to parasympathetic end of the spectrum, which is what we're after.

Once again, credit goes to Dr. John Rusin for putting this science together and turning it into a practical postworkout recovery technique. This is one of the most impactful recovery techniques I've experienced over the years, and if you're finding yourself in a highly stressed state (which happens to all of us at some point), you'll feel the difference immediately.

Method

1. Once your heart rate has decreased below about 90 beats per minute, remove your shoes, lie on your back and elevate your calves on a bench. Your hips and knees will be flexed at 90 degrees and your feet will be off the bench.

2. Close your eyes and turn your palms up to remove as much sensory stimulation as possible—especially from the sensitive areas of the palms of your hands and feet.

3. This is where diaphragmatic breathing comes into play, not for bracing, but for shifting from a sympathetic to a parasympathetic state. Although your breathing will start off at a faster pace, you'll want to work toward slowing your breath to 10 breaths per minute. It's not important that you actually reach this number, but it helps to guide the duration of each inhalation and exhalation.

4. Inhale through the nose and exhale through the mouth with pursed lips to help you to slow your breath and shift toward a calm alert state.

5. Maintain a positive attitude for the duration. Remember that the nervous system affects all, so think about the accomplishment of your workout and how great you're going to feel by applying this technique.

Bonus

1. Research in trained athletes has shown that this breathing practice combined with positive reflection (e.g., feeling great about your workout) and focus on the benefits of the program is an effective tool for CNS control and stress management (Dziembowska et al. 2016).

2. In addition to helping with the stresses of everyday life, this will help to optimize training performance and to reduce the risk of overtraining.

CNS RECOVERY

Another neural intervention relates to something that everyone needs—sleep. This is the time when your CNS recovers from the stresses of the day and "bakes in" what you've learned during the waking period. Unfortunately, it's so commonly disrupted that an entire industry has grown out of the consequences. If you're missing out on sleep, then your arm development and probably every aspect of your life is going to be compromised.

Whether it's due to an author's ability to reach beyond the pages, or just their terrible writing, you'll often find that reading about sleep can be a great cure for insomnia. For the sake of brevity we'll break it down to three actionable tips that my clients and I love, in order to help you get the sleep you need to adapt and perform optimally.

Blue Blockers

One of the most common sleep disruptors comes from blue-wavelength light, which destroys the natural sleep hormone melatonin—effectively telling our brain to wake up. Unfortunately, this is the main wavelength is that is emitted from the screens of electronic devices, including phones, laptops, and TVs. Trying to avoid all of these sources is a bit like trying to stop breathing, so we'll take the more practical approach. Wearing a cheap pair of orange tinted (nonprescription) glasses will help to filter out these wavelengths, as well as other ambient sources of light. As a throwback to the connection between light waves and recovery interventions discussed in chapter 2, you might think of this technique as orange shifting. Throw the glasses on for 60 to 90 minutes before your sleep time to maintain natural sleep-inducing melatonin levels.

The interventions presented in this chapter are all low-hanging fruit, but realistically not every single intervention is feasible for every person. In spite of that, putting on glasses before sleep is just about the easiest and least time consuming thing that you could do to improve your physique and performance. If you find yourself resistant to this practice in spite of the simplicity, it may be time to reevaluate.

Conditioning

Another simple technique is to develop a bedtime routine that will condition your body to prepare for rest. An example of this psychological conditioning is to consume your presleep meal followed by brushing, flossing, etc., then watching TV for 30 minutes before lights out. As a double win, I can tell you from five years of experience that donning orange glasses an hour or so before bed is a great environmental cue to shut down. Once the world "turns orange" to me, the unwinding process begins.

Belly Breathing

This is another excellent time to engage diaphragmatic breathing and the parasympathetic nervous system. It's a little different than your postworkout period during which you're trying to shift away from a highly stimulated sympathetic period of the lift. Before sleep, you should already be in a more parasympathetic state, with sensory deprivation coming in the form of darkness and quiet (or white noise). For this reason, it is more important to be as comfortable as possible (typically in your bed) and focus on diaphragmatic breathing.

Making Sleep Anabolic

A sleep-related fix that improves muscle growth from the nutritional side is related to one of the most common myths that refuses to die: sleep is your most anabolic time. In this case, **anabolic** refers specifically to the process of building muscle (the antonym is **catabolic**, the process of muscle breakdown). Although I believed this nocturnal anabolism myth for several years, my research experience once again helped to upgrade my thinking and subsequent application.

The idea was put to the test in a highly controlled lab setting called a general clinical research center (GCRC). In my case, this research center was a wing of a hospital manned by specially trained nurses and medical staff who were able to tightly control the environmental conditions, including nutrient intake, of our subjects. Because we were studying protein intake and **muscle protein synthesis** (the growth, recovery, and adaptation response), we needed strict enforcement of dietary restrictions. The actual studies always began very early in the morning, so our subjects would spend the preceding night sleeping under the watchful eye of the GCRC staff (to ensure dietary compliance).

After an overnight fast, we'd begin the morning study by playing the role of vampire and carefully extracting blood from the subjects' arteries. From this we could look at their levels of muscle anabolism, and without fail, the subjects were always in a state of muscle breakdown—in direct contrast to the anabolic myth.

The reason for the contradiction is simple: recovery and adaptation require both caloric energy and protein. When we're sleeping, we have neither. Worse yet, our vital functions still require these elements during this fasting time and readily break down our *de facto* store of protein (i.e., muscle) to meet their needs.

It's important to note that the sleep-is-anabolic myth in not simply incorrect, but it's the exact *opposite* of reality—our nightly sleep-induced fast is actually catabolic. So, by fixing this protein-fasted state, we're not only stopping the muscle breakdown, but we're fueling the muscle growth to actually make sleep anabolic. That's a double win that you can experience every single night.

One simple action is to consume a slowly digesting protein like milk-derived **casein**. This protein clots in the stomach and is slowly digested to provide a steady trickle of amino acids to the body. This will allow both your muscles and other tissues to be consistently fed throughout the night. Not only has this been shown to decrease muscle catabolism, but it turns your body into a 24-hour anabolic machine (Trommelen and van Loon 2016). Ingest 40 grams of slow protein before sleep if you are a lean 170-pound (77 kg) individual or roughly 1g protein for every 4 pounds (1.8 kg) of body weight. Specific timing isn't important, but the general idea is to consume the protein shortly before you retire as long as it doesn't disrupt sleep.

Casein powder is the easiest because the dose is precise, with minimal contribution of other calorie sources (fats and carbs). It is also the primary source that has been studied for this purpose. Alternatively, protein sources like lean red meats or whole eggs should suffice, but you will need to be aware of the caloric contribution of fats in these sources and adjust your daily intake accordingly.

Protein Pulse Feeding

Another important recovery intervention was discovered in the GCRC after the subjects consumed their first protein-containing meal of the day. Even if the subjects had never worked out a day in their lives, morning protein ingestion always caused a small activation of muscle growth. This anabolic effect is referred to as a **nutraceutical effect**, which is a direct biochemical change induced by a food or nutrient (Shimomura et al. 2006). In this case, it's the stimulation of muscle protein synthesis that you can take advantage of for growth, recovery, and adaptation.

To take advantage of this effect, one can consume a fast protein, which is quickly broken down into its component building blocks, called amino acids. I would suggest ingesting 25 grams of whey protein or 1 gram of protein for every 7 pounds (3.2 kg) of body weight when otherwise fasted. This can be repeated every two and a half to three hours. These amino acids are then absorbed into the bloodstream. An increase in the quantity of these amino acids in the blood serves as a signal to the muscle that it's being fed. This triggers the muscle to give the go-ahead to start building more (muscle) protein. That nutraceutical stimulation of muscle protein synthesis happens anytime amino acid levels in the blood start off relatively low and then are pulsed to a relatively high level. This **protein pulse feeding** means that once the amino acids (from ingested whey, in this example) are cleared from your bloodstream, you can repeat the process for another anabolic nutraceutical effect.

Whey protein isolate is ideal for this task because it is a highly purified form of this dairy-derived protein. Whey protein concentrate is slightly less pure and contains some remaining elements of the initial protein extraction from dairy products, such as the sugar lactose. Although both work well, whey protein isolate is more expensive. A commercial blend of both types is quite common and serves as an affordable compromise.

For an applied example, upon waking at 7 a.m., you consume 25 grams of protein with a granola bar containing 25 grams of carbohydrates. At 9:30 a.m., you consume another drink containing 25 grams of protein with 25 grams glucose as part of a feeder workout (see next section).

Based on the successful combination of research experience and client results, I initially published this applied theory in 2008 (Barr) and am excited to have had it validated by independent research four years later (Moore et al. 2012).

ACTIVE RECOVERY FEEDER WORKOUTS

This triple threat recovery technique combines nutrition and training to optimize your arm development, and it is going to be an incredibly rewarding experience (and a great time for you to take selfies). It begins by upgrading the following traditional theory for boosting recovery adaptation: increase blood flow to the muscle, which is thought to clear away biochemical waste and bring in more muscle-building nutrients (good stuff?). This appears to be at least half right, because the right combination of nutrients can alone stimulate blood flow, which conveniently facilitates their own delivery to cells. This accelerated transport is a powerful nutraceutical effect that is just waiting for another element to unlock its latent potential.

That element comes in the form of a specific type of exercise, and together, this becomes a potent combination. Although you can't isolate the increase in blood flow to specific muscles with food alone, you *can* do so by using **feeder workouts**. The result of combining the nutrient-stimulated blood flow with that caused by exercise is a massive pump, increased feeling of well-being, and accelerated recovery adaptation. We cap this system off with the final synergistic component: CNS recovery in the form of sympathetic shifting. Altogether the resulting protocol is referred to as a three-phase feeder workout.

Phase 1—Nutrition

The nutrition phase begins shortly before the workout (roughly 20-30 minutes prior depending on what's ingested). The combination of fast carbs and protein will stimulate blood flow, even before the exercise. Each of their more specific nutraceutical effects is mentioned in the list below.

How to. Consume a fast protein like whey to increase blood flow, stimulate muscle protein synthesis, and provide the amino acid building blocks to the muscle for repair and growth.

Example. Consume 25 grams of whey protein or 1 gram protein for every 7 pounds (3.2 kg) of body weight.

How to. Consume fast carbohydrates such as glucose or a sport drink to increase blood flow and fuel the exercise.

Example. Consume 25 to 40 grams, or 1 gram of carbs for every 4 to 7 pounds (1.8-3.2 kg) of body weight.

Phase 2—Contraction

The feeder workout is designed to further increase muscle blood flow (started by phase 1) and force-feed the muscle with the desired nutrients. This is accomplished by using concentric and isometric-focused exercise, such as sled training (discussed in chapter 7). A powerful cue is to imagine that this workout–nutrient combination is *forcing* the nutrients into every active muscle cell as you perform each rep. Sure, it's not scientifically accurate, but this cue really helps you to focus on squeezing during the concentric and isometric contractions, even if no load is present.

The key to the contraction phase of the feeder workout is to create a localized stimulation of blood flow but not cause further muscle damage or otherwise impair recovery adaptation.

Ideally this can be achieved through the use of bands or sled-based movements. Recall that sleds are used for recovery work because of the concentric-only nature of their movement. This means no damaging eccentric portion. The same can be said for bands when the eccentric portion is largely ignored. The band resistance at the lengthened portion of the eccentric rep, when more muscle microdamage can occur, is minimal. Also, unlike gravity-based loads, there's no momentum to worry about when allowing a fast eccentric movement with a band. For elastic resistance, you're just making sure that the band doesn't snap and hurt anyone. Think of it more as *guiding* the band back to its starting position rather than strictly controlling it. As an example, triceps push-downs can be performed concentrically and held isometrically, and then the band can be allowed to quickly return to starting position.

Biceps curls are a classic example of a feeder sled drag. With tension on the connector, the biceps are squeezed to flex the elbow against the sled resistance. The peak contraction is held for a moment, even after the sled has stopped moving or providing tension. No eccentric movement is performed, although you should win a prize if you can figure out how this would even be possible. Instead, the next rep is set up by returning your arms to the starting position of the concentric portion and walking away from the sled to create tension once again.

Repeat two similar exercises per body part from your last workout for three to four sets, each set lasting roughly 60 to 90 seconds, with 30 to 60 seconds of rest in between. The simplified objective here is really just to get a huge pump, so these parameters are offered as broad guidelines. As a result of this freedom, these workouts can be a lot of fun and provide a great opportunity for you to personalize according to your own preferences. Remember that the feeling here is to squeeze the muscle to force nutrients into your cells. This is intended to feed your muscle, not cause further mechanical stress.

For sled-based exercises, hold the peak contraction for a two-count before resetting for the next concentric part of the exercise.

One benefit of this low-intensity, low-duration exercise is that it allows you to perform other fitness-related modalities, during the same session, such as stretching and cardio. You can see examples of sled-based exercises to use in a feeder workout in chapter 7, Nontraditional Exercises.

SideBarr

Massage is commonly believed to facilitate recovery through increases in muscle blood flow. There are several problems with this idea, including the lack of definition for either massage (which is a broad category of diverse physical manipulation techniques) or recovery. Interestingly, research has shown that various types of massage do not increase muscle blood flow (Tiidus 2015). In my experience, presenting this evidence-based statement is consistently met with a negative emotional reaction, as though I am personally responsible for taking away something that people love. To be clear, this doesn't mean that your favorite type of massage isn't beneficial (because massages are *awesome!*); it simply means that the underlying mechanism does not seem to be blood flow related.

Phase 3—Sympathetic Shifting

With the contraction phase and any subsequent physical activity complete, you're going to be left with an incredibly rewarding pump. Even though you're not intentionally activating your sympathetic nervous system as you would for a standard lift, the ensuing sense of accomplishment makes the perfect time to facilitate neural recovery. Research shows that positive affirmation is a part of this recovery process, which means that piggybacking onto the great feeling you already have from the feeder workouts potentiates the effect. Speaking of positivity, don't forget to take selfies with your massive arm pump!

CREATINE MONOHYDRATE

We'd be remiss if we didn't explore the most effective and widely studied supplement on the planet, **creatine monohydrate**. I give credit to one of my personal mentors, Anthony Almada, for having introduced it to North America more than 30 years ago and letting me in on the secret that nothing beats creatine for enhancing arm muscularity and strength.

What Is It?

Creatine is a source of quick energy that naturally exists in every cell in the human body. We ingest it anytime we eat red meat, although you'd have to consume an excessive amount of beef to experience a performance- or physique-related benefit. The good news is that we have the supplemental form known as creatine monohydrate, which simply means that a water molecule is attached to that of creatine. Other types of creatine, which swap out the water with other molecules, have not been shown to be more effective than the inexpensive and widely studied monohydrate.

It's worth emphasizing that this discussion is simply a science-based overview for informational purposes and not a prescription or even a recommendation. For more information, you may want to consult with a licensed nutritionist who has either a sport specialization (such as a certified specialist in sports dietetics) or an advanced degree (e.g., master's or doctorate degree) in a biological science. These distinctions increase the likelihood that the individual will be familiar with the ingredient or capable of translating the research to application.

Is It Safe?

Research has consistently shown creatine monohydrate supplementation to be safe and effective in both healthy people and those in a variety of disease states (Kreider et al. 2017). Some people experience temporary gastrointestinal distress in the early days of creatine use. Although this is a short-lived phenomenon, it can often be avoided altogether by using smaller doses throughout the day.

The other so-called side effect is incredibly misunderstood and actually a big positive for us. It pertains to the fact that most of your cells are naturally filled with water, and this is especially true for muscle cells. Storing more water inside makes muscles look and feel like real muscle, because that's what *real* muscle is.

The level of muscle fullness can also be naturally manipulated by increasing your carbohydrate intake, for example. If you consume higher quantities of carbs for a short period of time (aka if you carb load), your muscles will store them within muscle as glycogen, and a lot more water along with it. This could actually create the appearance that you've quickly added an additional pound or two of solid muscle.

The misunderstanding about muscle hydration also applies to creatine use and the side effect referred to as water retention. People erroneously interpret the concept of water retention as bloating or water stored under the skin (which would look and feel like body fat). Importantly, the overwhelming majority of water storage accompanies creatine and glycogen inside of your muscle, which you'll quickly notice as fuller looking muscle (Kreider et al. 2017).

Storing more quick energy in the muscle (as creatine) helps to improve different types of performance, including muscle strength. Overall, this leads to more impactful workouts, which result in greater long-term muscle growth. Better yet, the water storage causes a rapid visible increase in muscularity but can also decrease the amount of natural muscle breakdown. The net result is, once again, more muscle.

Creatine is often dissolved in water and consumed at a dose of three to five grams per day in single or divided doses. The initial week of creatine use may consist of "loading," during which the muscle levels rapidly increase. This is accomplished using a total of 10 grams per day in divided doses. Excess creatine is simply excreted in urine, so there's no concern of overdose or more

SideBarr

Rapid weight loss during calorie-restricted and low-carb diets is caused by the excretion of this natural water storage in muscle, rather than actual fat loss. Anytime you consume insufficient carbohydrates, your body will burn through your stored carbs for energy and release the water along with it (ultimately excreted as urine).

This water loss is seen as rapid decreases in scale weight, but once there's no more glycogen and water to get rid of (usually in 4-7 days), the needle on the scale abruptly stops moving. Note: This water and glycogen storage also accounts for much of the initial weight rebound when a short-term dieter resumes their normal caloric intake.

specific long-term dosing protocols. The best way to avoid gastrointestinal distress is to begin with the lowest single dose of three grams and increase according to preference and tolerance.

WRAP-UP

This chapter has been a huge information dump, so you may need to use these very protocols to recover, starting right *now*. Although it takes a little time and practice to find how these techniques fit best into your lifestyle, you'll love the result. Remember that this personalization allows you to optimize your performance now but also allows you to adapt the techniques for years to come. This relentless, never-ending upgrade has already started for you, and this chapter in particular is intended to erase some of the outdated dogma about recovery. By replacing the mythology with current practices and a focus on adaptation, you're taking yet another giant leap ahead of the crowd. So be sure to unwind and get some sleep tonight, because your CNS has a lot of adaptive rewiring to do.

PART III

The Programs

Gym-Based Programming

You've exercised monastic patience to get through a ton of concepts, theories, and techniques, but now it's time to put them to work for you. This chapter incorporates the five key targets into a personalized training program that helps you to achieve maximum arm development. What makes this application even better is that instead of shoehorning the novel techniques into a traditional program, we'll upgrade the approach to programming, just as we did with everything else in this book. In order to do that, we'll first need to undo some of the damage engrained by traditional thinking and start with a clean slate. Rather than just read more words about it, this is something you'll need to experience through a helpful training challenge.

TARGETED GROWTH CHALLENGE

To help reinforce the importance of stimulation overload, we'll perform a simple experiment. Start with your favorite arm exercise and a load that you'd normally use for 8 to 12 reps. Drop that load by 20 percent for this single-set experiment. For example, if you normally use a 50-pound barbell for biceps curls, use 40 pounds for the test. Your goal is to perform a set with this lighter load and reach failure at the same repetition goal in under a minute (so no super slow reps). In this example, if you normally perform sets of eight reps with the 50-pound barbell, you want to do the same using 40 pounds, ensuring that by the end you couldn't perform another rep without cheating (i.e., you have reached muscular failure).

Test Summary
- Choose your favorite arm exercise.
- Drop the 8- to 12-rep training load by 20 percent.
- Perform a set to failure at the same rep goal (8-12), in less than one minute.

You may be surprised how easy it is for you to achieve targeted failure, even after dropping the weight by a massive 20 percent. In fact, you may not even reach the rep goal before your form breaks down. Either result is a big win, because it shows the depth of recruitment you can tap into when muscle stimulation becomes your focus, as opposed to simply throwing on (and then throwing around) load. Once you've experienced this breakthrough, you might question the effectiveness of other heavy sets that you've done in the past. This single example shows a fundamental problem with the chronic use of prescriptive loads based on percent repetition maximum (percent RM), which was introduced in chapter 1 (see consecutive contraction limit). The load itself doesn't matter as much as *how* you use it to stimulate your muscle.

Without overtly trying to do so, your success of this experiment is most likely achieved through the following:

1. Slowing the reps down (probably closer to a 2/1/1/1, resulting in a higher time under tension [TUT])
2. Maintaining strict technique (more tension on the muscle throughout, resulting in a higher TUT)
3. Internally focusing on squeezing your muscle (greater muscle inefficiency)

Altogether this offers a more pronounced and more thorough stimulation of metabolic growth and possibly even structural growth. Consider that we've spent time discussing each of the stimulus techniques you used, but you accomplished each of them organically by using only a single conceptual cue: *make the exercise harder.*

This intuitive achievement means that your body already knows how to do all of these things. The problem is that your body also wants to *not* do these things. It's up to you to override that primitive survival instinct and optimally stimulate your muscle to grow. This is where your **key performance indicators (KPIs)** come into play.

PROGRAMMING KPIS

One of the essential components of your optimized program is that it offers personal feedback and evaluation. This empowers you to continually assess how the plan is working and adjust accordingly. A generalized program may be somewhat effective in 90 percent of people, but *personal assessment is the key to taking your results to the next level.* We'll explore a few KPIs that you can use to evaluate your training stimuli and then make course corrections along the way to *deliver an experience that's custom tailored to you.*

Postworkout KPIs happen after your workout and are subdivided into short and long term. Short-term KPIs are used to evaluate the effect of your preceding workout, so you can adjust for your next lift. Long-term KPIs serve as a warning that your overall stress is too high, which could be due to excessive training volume or intensity.

KPIs that happen within the workout itself are referred to as **intraworkout**. They provide combined feedback about your previous lift as well as how you're performing on that day. As with postworkout KPIs, the goal is to use this information to refine your workout and achieve your biggest gains.

Delayed-Onset Muscle Soreness

The first short-term KPI consists of a relatively simple subjective evaluation of your delayed-onset muscle soreness (DOMS) in the days following your lift.

Muscle soreness is a result of the desirable microtrauma induced by the workout, which then triggers the body's immune system to start clearing away the damaged tissue and make room for new muscle. It's a bit like clearing out the debris from a construction site before starting the new, upgraded build. I appreciate that it's hard to make the word *trauma* seem innocuous, let alone desirable, even when prefaced with *micro*. But we can draw on the lesson of the recovery adaptation curve (chapter 2) to recognize that in this case, microtrauma is part of the stress stimulus (phase 1) that sets up the preadaptation phase (phase 2) for microtargeted structural growth (phase 4).

Thinking about this process as a connected chain of events also helps to explain why the soreness is delayed; it's a result of your body's initial identification of the damage, followed by a relatively slow immune and inflammation reaction. So, it's not the actual muscle damage that causes the pain, it's your body's delayed reaction to that damage (and it has nothing to do with lactic acid!).

When you experience greater DOMS than normal, it's a good sign that you've had a stronger training stimulus and are experiencing the proportionally amplified phase 2 effect. We saw an example of this, represented as a red shifted recovery adaptation curve in figure 2.2. Although the existence of DOMS is a good sign that growth has been induced, its absence does not suggest otherwise. There are two reasons for this, which also explain why we're not chasing soreness.

1. The response is highly individualized (some people almost never get sore).

2. It's more likely to occur after training with eccentric overload, for micro-targeted structural growth. This means that lifting to target metabolic hypertrophy is less likely to induce DOMS, which could make it harder to use as a KPI for this type of training.

Note that when you first use stimulation-focused training, you're likely to experience DOMS even though you're using lighter loads. This is because you're recruiting a greater proportion of your muscle fibers. Any previously untapped fibers will be unaccustomed to any training stimulus and will be very sensitive to anything you throw at it.

Distal Early Warning

When trying a new exercise, you want to watch out for excessive isolated DOMS that happens in smaller muscles that you didn't even know existed. This localized soreness means that you haven't trained these muscles, so they're taking a disproportionately high amount of stress stimulus. That concept was painfully hammered into me after a humbling (and hobbling) training experience. At the time, my leg workouts consisted of squatting to parallel with 455 pounds for sets of eight at a 2/1/2/1 tempo (TUT of 48 seconds), lying leg curls, and heavy cable leg adductions with an ankle attachment. This isn't intended as an attempt to impress, but to illustrate that my legs were used to dealing with heavy loads. As a lark, I trained with a friend at the local Y and decided to try the seated leg adductor machine (also known as [aka] the thigh squeezer, aka 'no' machine). I had never used this ridiculous machine before (I mean, *why would I?*), but I regularly trained this muscle group, so it wasn't a big deal to experiment for a couple of sets with a load that felt pretty light.

The result: in nearly three decades of lifting, I have never been that sore (before or since). The DOMS, isolated to my upper, inner thighs, impaired my ability to walk for four days. This happened because my usual cable adductor training focused the load at the ankle, while the machine placed the load at the knee. The resulting change in recruitment meant that muscles previously used only for support were now doing all of the work—and they got *wrecked*. This was an incredible lesson about the specificity of anatomically targeted training, as well as punishment from the training gods for my having scoffed at an exercise.

You can apply this lesson to your own training, based on the experiences of those who have used the programs herein. From this, be aware that you're most likely to experience this type of isolated soreness in your core (which is intentionally broad, but universally weak), your upper back (including shoulders), or your forearms. Whatever the case, if you experience a huge amount of isolated DOMS, use it as both a caution flag and an opportunity to better understand your body. Regarding the former, if a muscle group is bearing an unusually high amount of stress stimulus, it may be headed toward injury if pushed further. For example, if the only thing you feel from a new biceps exercise is an intense isolated forearm DOMS, you need to back off the load and let that muscle catch up to the others.

This is also a potentially exciting find, because it encourages you to evaluate your current training and figure out both *what* this isolated muscle is, and *why* it hasn't been activated before. That experience-driven personalization is one of the best ways to learn about your body's specific response to training.

Soreness is incredibly idiosyncratic, or widely variable between individuals, which makes it a very personal KPI. Some people rarely get sore while others start limping at the sight of a barbell. The key to this assessment is your *relative* soreness—are you more or less sore than you would be after a moderately hard workout?

Higher volume training, using greater loads, and especially eccentric-overload training, can all increase the magnitude of DOMS. The amount soreness you induce should progressively decrease as the muscle adapts week after week, so keep this in mind and adjust your weekly expectations of DOMS accordingly.

When you begin the program, you'll evaluate your level of soreness over the 24-hour following a lift. Although this is a highly variable subjective measure, during the first weeks of the program, you're looking for mild soreness and stiffness, especially at stretched positions. You can use the following two measurements as guides:

1. If you're too sore, wait to train the same muscle group until a minimum of 24 hours have passed after the soreness has dissipated.

2. If you're not feeling anything, reassess your training intensity. If you experience the same result and have evaluated the training parameters, add one set to each arm exercise. As a last resort, you may need to decrease the rep range and increase the load while maintaining rating of perceived exertion (RPE).

Localized Muscle Fatigue

Localized muscle fatigue is expected *during* the workout but should not be carried over from previous workouts. For example, your grip should not be limiting your barbell biceps curls, and core fatigue should not be limiting your goblet squat. How do you distinguish between localized muscle fatigue and DOMS? An example of localized muscle fatigue might be the feeling of "jelly" you get in your muscles toward the last set of a particularly grueling workout. You might find yourself tempted to take a shortcut in your reps, or loosen up your form, as a result of this feeling of weakness. By contrast, DOMS often manifests itself the morning (or subsequent mornings) after a particularly tough workout as a feeling of being rusted shut, accompanied by soreness or even pain in the affected muscles.

Due to the integrated nature of the human body, it is always important to be aware of your fatigue level in muscles that are indirectly targeted, such as shoulders, core, and those of the forearms and grip. This is useful both during the workout and in the hours and days following a lift. If this local muscle fatigue becomes limiting, adjust the program by reducing the volume of the implicated exercises.

One example of localized muscle fatigue could be in how you adjust your grip. If your grip becomes limiting, eliminate direct grip work and carries for at least one workout, until the problem resolves. Gradually reintroduce these exercises by starting with loaded carries once per week and reassess. As the simplest example of how to personalize your program based on KPI feedback, you can use the following guides: If limiting, reduce volume. When resolved, gradually reintroduce volume.

Systemic Fatigue

Systemic fatigue is a more serious long-term indicator, because it could be a sign of overtraining. This happens as a result of excessive stresses, both physical and psychological, so it's important to also be aware of environmental and lifestyle factors. These include things like stressful life events (e.g., exams, changing jobs, publisher deadlines, etc.), sleep deprivation, and inadequate nutrition.

You might experience systemic fatigue as an inability to fully wake up; ironically this is often accompanied by an inability to fall asleep (in spite of the fatigue). You may have brain fog, feel sluggish or run down, or you might experience any other descriptors for *always tired*.

Ironically, one of the best ways to help alleviate some of this stress is physical activity, although it's typically the last thing you want to do during these periods. Most often, the key is that the activity is low intensity and enjoyable—you're not trying to set personal records during this time.

If you can rule out lifestyle factors and external stresses but the fatigue persists, it's time to take an unplanned break from training. Start with one week completely off of lifting and reassess. If you're feeling refreshed and eager to train again, you'll likely come back with increased strength and physical performance. There's nothing magical about a seven-day period, so if you find that you need more time off, be sure to take it. If the systemic fatigue persists after a layoff, you may want to consult a medical professional.

Mood State

Mood state offers another long-term indicator, from which prolonged disturbances will usually imply a necessary reduction in training volume. These disturbances could be everything from a lack of motivation to train all the way up to depression. This subjective feeling of being burned out may come with the physical component of chronic fatigue, but the symptoms are idiosyncratic, which makes it more challenging to identify. Disturbances in mood state are most common in hard-training athletes who perform excessive volume without enough rest.

The good news is that this KPI is simple to identify, and even small changes could be detected before they become more serious. You might even notice the mood changes on your own. Additionally, there are various psychological tests that can be taken, such as the profile of mood states (POMS). These tests are simple, effective, free, and widely available. Finally, tests like the POMS can be used for personal assessment but become even more informative when externally reviewed, typically by a coach or personal trainer.

Intraworkout KPIs

Along with gravity-restricted training, the one-repetition maximum (1RM) and subsequent prescriptive loading (percent 1RM) have achieved the exercise equivalent of **brand annihilation**. This is the marketing term applied when a specific brand name comes to represent an entire product category, such as referring to all facial tissue as Kleenex (which is a trademarked brand name for a specific product). Similarly, the 1RM seems to be the only game in town when it comes to evaluating your training or progression.

Despite their ubiquity, general programs based on percent RM load seems to imply clairvoyance—they predict how you'll respond, and they use strength

---

SideBarr: Time Travel Revelation

The KPI upgrade is one of many inspired by engineer and cofounder of Keiser equipment, Dennis Keiser. He blew my mind with a friendly and enlightening challenge that I now pose to you:

"Think about your life today and try to imagine what it would have been like 100 years ago. Which aspects would be the same, and which would be different?" (Dennis Keiser, pers. comm.).

The simple answer is that nearly everything would be different—*profoundly* so. As a result, any similarities you could retain are exceptional and noteworthy. If you couldn't think of any, which is common and acceptable, here's the punch line: in spite of the endless differences, your training would be incredibly similar to what it is today, if not identical.

Think about that. Of all the changes in the past century, your training would not be one of them. Now consider that although barbells, dumbbells, and kettlebells existed even back then, you could take your time-traveling DeLorean (or TARDIS) back further and still find gravity-based loads to use for exercise. This ranges from using rocks and dinosaurs as resistance, to body-weight calisthenics and even cardio (e.g., running away from the dinosaur that you just tried to lift).

I should warn you that the more you think about this, only to find that training with gravity resistance might be the only consistent thread throughout, the more mind-blowing this idea becomes.

This is why the exclusive use of gravity loads (aka iron) and percent RMs reflect what is known as **Iron Age thinking** and **Iron Age training** (aka dinosaur training).

as the defining parameter. But after our dissection of the targeted anatomy of a rep (in chapter 1) and the importance of muscle stimulation (chapter 2), it may be easier to see why prescribing exercise using a predetermined percent of your maximum is also incredibly limiting. Let's explore this critical point so you can add programming to your list of massive upgrades (to give you massive arms).

We've spent so much time dissecting and upgrading the five key targets concepts (related to training and stimulating muscle growth) that it would be surprising, if not overtly hypocritical, if we couldn't do the same for our programming progressions. After all, the traditional prescription and progression via percent RM is completely reliant on both gravity-based loads and the limits of the concentric rep. It also fails to take into account the individual differences for both training stimuli and for subsequent adaptive responses.

Worse yet, using a weekly increase in percent RM to both predict *and* measure progress feeds the parasite that is our ego. Erroneously, this translates into the thinking, and then practice, that more weight is better. So, in addition to the perceived progress of adding weight (i.e., numbers going up), we're psychologically programmed by our ego to feel better about ourselves by lifting more. This happens irrespective of *actual* measurement or progress and leads to the loosey goosey training technique that you find every time you walk into a gym. Surely, we can do better.

KPI UPGRADE—RPE

A more effective KPI would need to overcome many of the restrictions encountered with percent RMs, apply to a broader range of resistance types, and offer greater personalization. Better yet, we'll use a real-time KPI that does the following:

- It works with traditional gravity-based loads, sets, and reps.
- It works with different types of nongravity resistance, like bands.
- It works across different contraction types and ROMs.
- It promotes functional stimulation rather than excessive weight.
- It is personalized to your weekly progress.
- It is personalized to the workout day itself.

Given the hyperbole that the fitness industry is infamous for, you might be thinking, "So much [sic] upgrades? But David, that's unpossible [sic]!" But this "magical" KPI is nothing more than your own effort, which we've seen expressed as **rating of perceived exertion (RPE)** (chapter 2). You'll use the 10-point RPE scale or a 0 to 100 percent effort scale to evaluate how hard you're working and make changes as needed, even within the workout. Although it may be a bit of a stretch to think of effort as a KPI, it fits our broad definition of personalized feedback used to affect training.

Generally speaking, this type of real-time evaluation and adjustment is known as **autoregulation**—the use of personal feedback to adjust your training to your abilities on that day. You might think of it as training by feel. This technique provides a level of specificity, not only for each individual, but also within each workout.

For example, everyone has a day when they feel off of their game. Whether it's due to a lack of sleep, poor nutrition, or just general psychological stress, this common occurrence will affect your workout. Using RPE allows you to tailor your load to this suboptimal state, ensuring that your workout is optimal for that day.

One potential downside happens due to the subjective nature of relative intensity. This means that the concept of *hard* will be different among individuals, resulting in some people pushing themselves too much, while others won't push at all. In my experience, the latter is common with children, while *you* are more likely to drift toward the former.

This prospective issue has been addressed by an expert in this area, Dr. Eric Helms, using a technique called **anchoring**. This is the process of standardizing intensity among individuals. In your case, you'll establish this anchor by completing a set to failure, so you'll really know what an RPE of 10 feels like.

Reps in Reserve

Autoregulation works cohesively with another research-based method first introduced to me by Dr. Mike Israetel, called **reps in reserve** (**RIR**; Helms et al. 2016). This is an estimation of how many reps you have left in the tank when you complete a set. For example, if you perform a set of 10 reps with moderate-high intensity, you might feel like you are able to perform 2 more before failure. This would mean that you performed the set with two RIR.

RIR = estimated maximum reps – chosen number of reps

As with effort, RIR may not traditionally be thought of as a KPI, but it checks the boxes for personalized feedback and training impact. You'll organically develop your skill to predict RIR along with that of RPE, which makes it a natural adjunct with autogenic training. Eventually, you'll be able to predict how many reps you can perform with a given load, just by feel. Note that the greater your effort during a set, the fewer reps you'll have left in the tank. This RPE and RIR relationship is illustrated in table 9.1. The RPE of 10 reflects maximal intensity (aka 100 percent intensity) and momentary muscular failure, such that no further reps could be performed with full ROM and tight form (aka zero RIR).

The six KPIs are summarized for quick reference in table 9.2.

Table 9.1 Crossover Between RPE and RIR Scales

RPE	RIR
10	0
9	1
8	2
7	3
6	4
5	5

Table 9.2 Summary of KPIs

Postworkout	
Short-term	**Long term**
DOMS	Systemic fatigue
Muscle fatigue	Negative mood state
Intraworkout	
Relative effort	RPE
Anticipated actions	RIR

Test With 100 Percent Failure Rate

As with every other component of arm training, the more you use this skill, the better you become (Ormsbee et al. 2019). So, despite the name, there's no pass or fail here—the test is all about developing your personalized skill in assessing RIR and anchoring maximal RPE. The early objective is to get the feel of muscle fatigue and RPE as you approach momentary muscular failure (RIR = 0).

Imagine that you want to assess your RIR on triceps push-downs. Based on your experience, you estimate that you can perform a maximum of 12 reps with 55 pounds (25 kg; i.e., you could not perform a 13th rep with tight form). If you're trying to stop the set with an intensity of two RIR, you'd be performing 10 reps with this load. After a first work set, you can increase the fidelity of this estimate through an assessment (by going to failure). This will provide the feedback from which you establish your RIR during the next workout.

So, if you estimate a 12-rep max but hit failure at 10 reps, you've only *slightly* overestimated your RIR. If, on the other hand, you performed 15 reps, you've *under*estimated your RIR and will want to increase the load to maintain perceived intensity.

Importantly, assessment is all about providing you with personalized information that no one else can give you. Remember, the point is to organically upgrade your skill; it's not about being right or wrong. Just as with exercise technique, even the most advanced lifters on the planet are continually developing this skill.

At most, this test can be conducted once weekly, outside of deload and off weeks. Also, you can record yourself during these sets to ensure that your form on the final maximal effort rep, is nearly identical to that of the first. The anchor is at zero RIR, so as we move farther away from the point of failure, our ability to accurately predict RIR decreases. For this reason, increasing RIR beyond five is not advised for work sets. If lighter intensity is employed for a deload, then there's no need to use RIR.

SideBarr: Is Perfect Form Perfect for You?

From experience, I can tell you that maintaining rigorous exercise technique, proper breathing and bracing, momentum-free movement, and intensely focused muscle contraction on every rep might be effective, but it's *exhausting*. So, although we want to initially find our personalized ideals for each rep (to learn the movement and the RIR, for example), the resulting high RPE ensures that it is not a realistic long-term training plan.

One reason is that you'll have new elements to focus on during new exercises, and each has an initial energetic cost that raises RPE. This isn't a problem, but it is something to be aware of during execution and subsequent evaluation. Although the early training blocks require a significant amount of mental energy, this is a short-term investment that will be overwhelmingly worth your while.

As we come to appreciate maximal muscle contraction, newfound core strength, and so on, they will start to become automatic, so we'll be able to slightly relax the intensity of our focus on these elements. This decreases the overall intensity of the workout and often comes as a welcome reprieve.

Lastly, it is important that you develop a baseline understanding of what strict form feels like throughout the ROM, so you know to what extent you may be deviating as you fatigue. When you become very proficient, you can do so strategically (e.g., using a little momentum after the final concentric to perform an extra exaggerated eccentric rep). This type of reality injection is an effective way to maintain long-term workout effectiveness and enjoyment.

PRINCIPLE OF PROGRESSION

Different training parameters provide different levels of growth stimuli between individuals. Some people have muscle that is best stimulated by high TUT (e.g., high reps and lighter load), while others by heavier loads and minimal fatigue. Even when an ideal stimulus is used, the subsequent magnitude of adaptive response (e.g., amount of resulting growth and strength) differs between people.

Rather than feeling overwhelmed by this and experiencing paralysis by analysis, know that this is where the art and science of programming synergize. It is with this awareness that we need to start with generalized training templates. By striking a balance between following a template and adjusting based on your own training response, you'll set yourself up for much greater success.

Getting Started

In spite of the limits, there's no getting around the use of load-based progressions while you feel your way through the program. But instead of relying on load alone, you'll use the upgrades in your KPI toolbox to refine your training and develop your skills.

Begin with a load-based progression and record RPE on each set. Adding a video of the set can provide feedback about prospective underestimation. For example, imagine that you record an RPE of seven after a set of triceps extensions. But during video playback, you see that there's so much hip flexion and extension throughout, that you initially mistake the exercise for a Romanian deadlift. This is a great indicator that you need to drop the load, reestablish the feeling of tight form, and reevaluate your RPE.

It must be reemphasized that you'll have far better results when you focus on developing your training skills (e.g., bracing, establishing RPE, etc.), rather than trying to progress by simply throwing on weight.

The desired rep limit decreases a little each week, which allows you to establish the feel for each exercise across a small change in load. On average, this will result in a 5 to 10 percent weekly increase in load. Note that your RPE also increases each week, which develops your familiarity with higher intensity. By the end of the first training block, you'll perform the final set of each exercise to failure. This provides a strong training stimulus and allows you to anchor maximal intensity.

As a final reminder, if the training volume or frequency ever seems excessively high or inadequately low as shown in the template, that perception is merely an artifact of traditional programming*. You control every aspect of the stimulus based on the insights gleaned from your KPIs. So, if you need more or less of any parameter (such as sets per exercise), you have the power to make these changes and personalize your training blueprint.

This double meaning of 'programming' refers to a training plan, as well as cognitive inculcation.

Rational Program Structure

The program is organized by different levels of time, and you'll find it easier to take in if you use the summary tables 9.3 and 9.4 to follow along with the written description. The broadest period is a mesocycle or phase, which is a general description of the program goal. For example the mesocycle in table 9.4 is the metabolic hypertrophy foundation phase.

This mesocycle lasts for 10 total weeks and consists of two training blocks, each concluded with a deload or rest week. The training blocks themselves are composed of five microcycles—one per week. The weekly microcycle consists of two workouts per muscle group, simply called day 1 and day 2. Week 5 of phase 1 is a deload week, during which volume and intensity are reduced, and week 10 is a complete active rest week.

Metabolic Hypertrophy Foundation Program

This is the most important phase of your program because it establishes the baseline for the rest of your training. Stated differently, this is where your personalized training domination begins. It is here where you practice your new skills, get the feel of new exercises, establish your training loads, and start to evaluate your specific needs (based on KPIs).

When establishing week 1 intensity (RPE), aim for a load that will allow you to perform about 15 reps. If assessed correctly, this will start off feeling light but should become challenging by the end of each set. Perform up to 12 reps per set, as long as you feel like you could perform more. If, by rep 12, you feel like you could keep going past 15, reassess your internal tension and locus of focus. When you are confident that you've optimized this, add weight.

Table 9.3 The Metabolic Hypertrophy Foundation Program Overview

Sets per exercise	3
Exercises per arm group	3
Tempo (TUT)	2/0/1/0
Interset rest	2 min

Table 9.4 The Metabolic Hypertrophy Foundation Program

Mesocycle	Metabolic hypertrophy foundation									
Block	Block 1					Block 2				
Microcycle or week	1	2	3	4	5	6	7	8	9	10
Reps	12	10	8	8	Deload	12	10	8	8	Off
RPE	6-7	7-8	8	8-10*	Deload	6-7	7-8	8	8-10*	Off

*The last set of each arm exercise is performed to failure.

Table 9.5 Workouts Within a Microcycle

Monday	Tuesday	Wednesday	Thursday	Friday	Saturday	Sunday
Biceps day 1	Triceps day 1	Off or recovery work	Biceps day 2	Triceps day 2	Off or recovery work	Off
Barbell curl (p. 148)	Bench press (p. 88)		Preacher curl (p. 130)	Banded push-up (p. 94)		
Reverse lunge (p. 64)	Suspension high-elbow row (p. 74)		Bulgarian split squat (p. 66)	Pull-down, pull-up (p. 78)		
Cable flex curl (p. 146)	Seated overhead extension (p. 96)		Incline dumbbell curl (p. 152)	Overhead rope (p. 108)		
Cable fly (p. 70)	Goblet squat (p. 54)		Kettlebell press (p. 72)	Quad-focused squat (p. 56)		
X-body hammer curl (p. 164)	Pit stain press (p. 98)		Pronated barbell curl (p. 161)	Supinated extension (p. 102)		
Ball hamstring curl (p. 62)			Suitcase carry (p. 80)			

With exercises for the six foundational movement patterns, maintain the approximate rep scheme but throttle your intensity to 70 to 80 percent so that you can focus your efforts on your arm exercises. The exercises are broken down by workout within a microcycle, shown in table 9.5.

Week 5 (Deload)

This is an active recovery week that will be very helpful after the week 4 microcycle. Perform sets of 10 reps with about half the load used in week 4. As a literal change of pace, the tempo of each rep can be increased.

Block 2

This second block of phase 1 is identical to the first block with a couple of notable exceptions. Your loads will be slightly greater having progressed through block 1. Perform the last rep of each arm exercise with a three-second eccentric portion. This will help you develop a little more muscle toughness. Lastly, rather than a deload after the first four weeks, the final week is completely off to recharge your batteries for your next program.

Your next training phase can repeat the first two blocks while experimenting with different exercises, intensities, and so on. As an advanced alternative, a strength phase can be performed, which provides different stimuli and might serve a refreshing change. This phase is added in advanced programming.

WRAP-UP

Along with building muscle, you've also developed a huge knowledge base from the preceding chapters. As you synthesize that information, you'll see that this chapter offers the next organic steps: programming and personalized KPIs. Developing the skills of personal awareness from using these KPIs comes with the gift of becoming more in tune with both your mind and body. This effect is enhanced when used in conjunction with the hypertrophy training template, which collectively serves as a quick start guide. By the time you're through the program, you'll have acquired the tools to turn any training template into your own personalized blueprint for muscle construction.

Limited-Equipment Training

If you've ever been stranded on a desert island, trapped in the past because of a temporal paradox, or isolated due to a pandemic, you've experienced the challenges that come with limited equipment options. But even if you can't yet relate there will come a time when you are forced to train with limited equipment, during which it may seem as though stimulating muscle growth is an impossible task. This is especially true of you're used to lifting in a commercial gym with every conceivable tool at your disposal. But *there are surprising advantages to limited-equipment training*. In fact, I recommend that all clients adopt a limited-equipment program for two weeks (bare minimum) at least once a year.

There are *at least* three benefits you'll experience from doing so:

1. Physical and psychological freedom
2. Long-term physical preparedness and resilience
3. Peak muscle activation

Even if used for a short time, each of these benefits will help to improve subsequent gym workouts and your overall physique development. Let's take a closer look to see how limited-equipment training can be a huge benefit to you.

PHYSICAL AND PSYCHOLOGICAL FREEDOM

We may get into a groove with training, which can creep into a habit of doing the same things over and over. This breeds complacency, and what began as smooth progress becomes a rut. What once served as guide rails turn into walls, and we find ourselves stuck. All too often, it is only when forced from our groove that we resort to novelty and innovation.

We've beaten to death the limits we impose with concentric exercises, gravity-based loads, and percent RM–based progressions. And with limited equipment, they've all gone out the window. What, dear reader, are we to do about it? Hint: If you've read the nine preceding chapters, you may already know.

In answering, it may seem as though the entire purpose of this book has been to set you up for success in this one chapter. Adopting a broader perspective reveals that limited-equipment training is only one scenario you can encounter, but *the principles established in the preceding chapters empower you to be prepared for any situation.*

Before continuing, we have to pause for a moment to appreciate the irony. By limiting our training options, we actually experience the freedom from our long-established cognitive and physical constraints.

LONG-TERM PHYSICAL PREPAREDNESS AND RESILIENCE

Limited-equipment training helps you get in touch with your core, and proactively fix weak points you probably didn't know you had. This powerful concept was best illustrated to me by Pain Free Performance Specialist Certification (PPSC) Chief Operating Officer Clifton Harski, who suggests that our natural inclination toward training our strengths is like developing a callus on your hand. Just as our muscle becomes stronger with training, a callus is an adaptation of our skin, which becomes thicker and more protective against localized friction (e.g., at the base of our fingers). This natural response is great for specific stimuli, but when we apply novel stresses outside of our adapted range, damage can result, even if those stresses are relatively small compared to what we're used to handling within our usual range.

For example, calluses don't rip at their thick center, but around the weaker outside portion where the adaptation *hasn't* occurred. The same adaptive specificity can happen with training. As a simple example, consider the typical gym member who executes the barbell bench press with only the upper one third of range of motion (ROM). He may become quite well adapted to this upper portion of the movement, but when he moves outside this range (intentional or not), his body has no idea what's going on. Because he lacks the structural or neural adaptations to allow for this ROM when loaded, he loses control and ends up stapled to the bench.

This is probably the simplest of many examples to illustrate adaptive specificity using different training parameters. To appreciate the breadth of this rabbit hole, you may also recognize the hubris of performing a light but novel thigh adductor exercise and experiencing days of pain as a result (chapter 9). A final example happens during situations when you need to react quickly, such as when slipping on ice while walking your small dog, stepping on a small dog bone, sitting on a small dog toy, or tripping on a small dog.

There are even situations not related to small dogs in which you may need to react quickly, and it is the breadth of your physical preparedness that will help you come through unscathed.

It may seem as though we're exceptionally arm-focused herein, but we're really establishing the guiding principles that will help you develop long-term resilience, health, and physique development. The previous examples help to illustrate why achieving this long-term goal requires you to train the body with a multitude of different exercises, loading patterns, ROMs, and so on. This shouldn't seem daunting but perceived as an opportunity to keep things interesting, have fun, and learn.

PEAK MUSCLE ACTIVATION

Training with limited equipment helps you get in touch with your peak muscle contraction. You can think of this as acquiring the skill to develop maximal muscle contraction across different exercises. The way to do this is called the **full flex method**, and you might recognize it as an exaggerated version of the intrinsic locus of focus (key 5).

In brief, you'll develop the skill of maximal muscle recruitment to facilitate the rest of your muscle stimulation. Begin following preworkout activation and a warm-up set (or two) of an exercise. Perform a light or completely deloaded rep that allows you to hold the peak contracted phase (at the end of the concentric movement, before beginning the eccentric movement). Your goal is to identify and squeeze your working musculature as hard as possible. Imagine that you're on stage and trying to pose in front of hundreds of people—that's the level of contraction you're after.

The more you practice this, the harder you'll be able to contract and the more fibers you'll recruit. Also, you'll come to identify how subtle tweaks in contraction can activate muscles differently. This method works especially well for recognizing what the hell is happening during exercises that involve numerous active muscles, like a pull-up. The goal is to progressively improve your ability to execute these peak contractions while using heavier loads to better stimulate muscle growth. This full flex method helps to increase the challenge during limited-equipment training, which you'll see implemented in the upcoming body-weight program.

OPTIMIZE ECCENTRIC MOVEMENTS

Traditionally, having access to limited equipment would make it slightly more challenging for you to induce structural growth. This is an easy fix because you'll provide high-force stress stimuli to your arm musculature by emphasizing elastic resistance-based eccentric overload techniques. The following tips will help you to implement eccentric training and take advantage of your full growth potential.

Use the Top 50 Percent of Your Full ROM

Eccentric contractions are infamous for causing muscle damage and delayed-onset muscle soreness (DOMS), which you know better as growth stimulation. The more lengthened the muscle as it's undergoing eccentric loading, the greater the damage. Eventually, this can be a powerful stimulus, but it's easy to overdo it. When starting out, it doesn't take much to damage or stimulate muscle. For this reason, begin by using eccentric overload in the shortest 50 percent of the eccentric ROM, right after the concentric portion of the rep. Once proficiency is gained with these techniques and a good deal of muscle toughness against eccentric damage has developed, this can be extended to two thirds of the full ROM.

Use the Two-Up, One-Down Technique

You'll use two limbs for the concentric part of an exercise, but the entire eccentric load is handled by one. For example, perform the concentric part of a two-handle cable biceps curl using both arms. Execute the subsequent eccentric with one arm while the other spots. Another example is the banded triceps push-down, in which one hand grasps the low point inside of a high-anchored band with an overhand (pronated) grip. The other hand will help to stretch the band to full elbow extension (i.e., perform the concentric part of the movement), and if more tension is desired, body weight can help stretch the band farther with both arms holding this locked elbow position. The working arm then performs a one-arm eccentric movement.

Use Band-Specific Techniques

Elastic resistance provides more opportunities to create an eccentric overload on your arm musculature. For example, you can establish the end concentric position of an exercise while there is minimal tension on the band. By stepping away from the anchor point and lengthening the band, you can greatly increase tension for the eccentric portion of the rep. As an example, you begin the eccentric overloaded one-arm row by performing the concentric movement close to the anchor, so that there is no tension on the band. While holding the peak contraction position (supported by the nonworking arm), you progressively step away from the anchor to stretch the band, until the tension becomes much higher than could be realized through a traditional concentric rep. The support arm is then removed, and the eccentric row is resisted by the working arm.

Stabilize As Much As Possible

If you've seen anyone squirm while performing a heavy bench press, you'll know that your whole body may want to get involved when fighting a heavy load. This is especially true when you're getting used to the novel feeling of trying to contract against a load that's overwhelming you (in spite of your efforts). For maximal effectiveness, you want to minimize body movement and maintain focus on the muscle by stabilizing your body as much as possible. For example, along with bracing your core, your shoulder and arm can be further stabilized by using the shoulder-lock technique. You might recognize this as a reiteration of stabilizing tension from key 5, and its exaggerated importance when using eccentric overload is warranted.

It's worth emphasizing that this is one of the reasons that arm-specific training really helps eccentric overload to shine. The isolated nature of these movements minimizes the number of joints needed for stability, which you'll come to appreciate when performing these high-tension exercises. As an example, consider how little eccentric overload you could apply during a single leg squat. In contrast, perform the same mental exercise with a concentration curl. It should be clear that greater stability allows for a more productive eccentric overload.

Use Cluster Training

Unlike traditional sets that use consecutive repetitions to induce fatigue (remember the con-con-lim), eccentric overload training emphasizes the amount of force produced during individual reps. For this reason, it is best to use **cluster training**, in which a brief rest (e.g., a few seconds) is taken between each pair of reps. Alternating arms with each rep is another option for minimizing the reduction in force output you experience as your muscle fatigues, while also improving efficiency (i.e., less overall workout time). The result is that you'll have maximal strength available for each rep (i.e., more force = more gains).

PULL-UP PROGRESSIONS
FOR LOADING ADJUSTMENTS

Not only is the pull-up a great exercise overall, but it ties together the elements of this chapter: body weight, band training, and eccentric overload. You've seen the pull-up, pull-down technique description, but the available progressions give the perfect opportunity to showcase this common exercise.

Progression 1—Banded Assistance

As a progression, bands can be looped from the overhead bar (or wherever you grip) and one of your knees placed through the hanging loop. This will provide progressively greater assistance, rather than resistance, as you descend. When you begin to pull up, you may opt to accelerate your body weight from the bottom, taking advantage of the assistance the stretched elastic provides out of the hole. This is helpful for reaching the challenging top portion of the exercise.

Progression 2—Body-Weight Eccentric Movement

A full body-weight eccentric movement or two can be added as a final cluster set once the banded sets are complete. This gives the feel of the full unassisted movement and a lot of muscle growth stimulus. Note that DOMS may be significant the first time this is done but should be greatly reduced in magnitude each time it is performed.

For the unassisted eccentric position, you will use your legs to get into the top position using a rack, bench, or other apparatus. After establishing the peak contracted (i.e., starting position) with your upper body, you can remove your first supporting leg and then the other, to ensure stability (i.e., no swaying). This is similar to the way in which you step back with one leg at a time to stabilize your body for a push-up.

Jumping pull-ups, in which you try to establish starting position by jumping into place, are a suboptimal last resort because they don't allow you to establish a stable peak contraction before performing the eccentric.

Progression 3—Added Load

As a final progression, more overload can be provided by attaching a plate to a weight belt, through the use of a hanging support chain. It can be a difficult position to set up, but I've found that initially having slack in the loaded chain helps you to set your hands with the correct placement, so you can then use your lower body to get into starting position.

As an alternative, a dumbbell may be between your knees when they are flexed at 90 degrees. It allows you to support a dumbbell between your upper calves, although it requires a spotter to place and remove.

BARE BONES BODY-WEIGHT TRAINING

Whether you're a calisthenic-inspired body-weight enthusiast or just want to mix up your workout, switching to body-weight training will give your brain and body the refreshing changes they need.

The best support of bare bones body-weight training comes from one of my greatest training influencers and owner of ClaytonFit.com, Nick Clayton:

> *Bodyweight training is a golden opportunity often missed by gym rats, because it's one of the most efficient ways to improve total body strength, coordination, and stability. The result is a noticeable carryover to your physique and subsequent performance, both in and out of the gym (Nick Clayton, pers. comm.).*

Body-weight training is traditionally more focused on the strength and skill of calisthenic movements, rather than pure muscle hypertrophy. You can probably think of male gymnasts with huge arms, which helps sell the benefit, just as the physique of a pro bodybuilder helps to sell supplements. But in our reality, it's important to recognize that the physiques of the genetic elite were not the result of an optimized arm-training program. We did not win the genetic lottery, so we have to train smarter.

Although a great deal of muscle can be developed in this way, body weight has limitations, particularly when it comes to arm-specific hypertrophy. As an example, the limited ability to load a push-up might mean that this exercise is useless for developing massive arms. For a welcome rebuttal, consider the SideBarr.

SideBarr: The High Rep Heresy

Witnessing history can be a great experience even if observed from the sidelines. In this case, I happened to be moderating what was to become a landmark presentation at a personal training conference. During the talk, the presenter had the audacity to suggest that high-rep training (25-35) was as effective as lower rep training (8-12) for muscle growth. This statement was clearly heretical, because at the time everyone "*knew*" that 8 to 12 was *the* rep range for growth. Following the presentation, a palpable unease permeated the audience as they performed the mental gymnastics to refute the blasphemous information and maintain the comfort of the status quo. During that time (which can only be described as the stunned silence), you could almost imagine the faint echo of pitchforks being sharpened and cries of, "He's a witch! He turned me into a newt!"

Although the paradigm shift was initially met with psychological resistance, the credibility of the speaker won the day. The talk was delivered by noted hypertrophy expert Dr. Brad Schoenfeld, whose research contributions and training book, *The M.A.X. Muscle Plan,* have repeatedly inspired this very work. Further, on that day he was not merely spouting his subjective opinion, but rather presenting objective data (Schoenfeld et al. 2015).

Observing those data through a lens of precision microtargeting (key 4), we can interpret the result as high reps created a greater metabolic stimulus, at the expense of structural growth. As a takeaway, you can find comfort in knowing that even with little equipment, high-rep training will give you results. Better yet, we'll make the training-induced metabolic stress more time efficient for you *and* forgo any compromise by including an eccentric emphasis for structural growth.

PROGRAM 1: THE BODY-WEIGHT PROGRAM

Because of their brief duration and high rating of perceived exertion (RPE), the arm exercises are performed at the beginning of a body-weight session or as their own separate arm training day (table 10.1).

Option 1: If these exercises are added to a body-weight workout, choose either biceps or triceps exercises, saving the other muscle group for the next session.

Option 2: If you're performing a full arm-specific training day, swap out the modified muscle-up for triceps walks. Otherwise, the carryover between pull-ups and muscle-ups will limit your strength potential on both.

This workout puts you in the driver's seat for dictating load and intensity. Each exercise can be modified to offer some assistance during the concentric phase, so that the resistance approximates a 15RM, while the eccentric movement is performed for two seconds by minimizing this assistance. The description of pull-up progressions shows an example of how resistance can be decreased or increased, based on your needs.

There's no objective measure of load, so RPE, total repetition number, and your subsequent DOMS will dictate arm training volume. Intense contractions are emphasized, and the goal is to complete the number of repetitions within the given time frame, rather than performing traditional consecutive reps and sets. This means that if you need to take a 10-second break after a rep, you should do so. Start with an RPE of six and progressively increase for two weeks based on resulting DOMS and familiarity with the exercises. As you become stronger and more skilled with each exercise, you'll organically develop the accompanying skill of precisely dictating RPE.

Week 1: 10 total reps per exercise, within two min, RPE of six

Week 2: 15 total reps per exercise, within three min, RPE of seven

Week 3: 20 total reps per exercise, within four min, RPE of eight

The week refers to calendar week, irrespective of your training frequency. This means that the same repetition goal is used for every arm-training set, whether you're performing it once or three times that week.

Table 10.1 Arm-Specific Body-Weight Workout Overview

	Day 1	**Day 2**
Exercise 1	Nilsson curl (p. 140)	Modified muscle-up (p. 100)
Exercise 2	Pull-up	Tiger bends (p. 106)
	Nonarm movements	Nonarm movements
Finisher	Rice bucket (p. 210)	Push-up

The frequency of this training is dictated by your key performance indicator of soreness, which means that it can occur as frequently or infrequently as you need. For example, if you don't feel anything after your first workout, you can perform again two days later and increase the load on the eccentric portion. Conversely, if you find yourself too sore and need a week off, back off the eccentric loading. As you discover your response to each exercise, remember that it's better to start with less intensity and progressively ramp up each workout, rather than go too hard out of the gate and be sore for a week.

There are two notable exceptions to the repetition scheme, each of which is performed at the end of the workout.

1. Rice bucket work will finish off your grip using two sets of 30 seconds (each arm).

2. Push-ups will use the same number of repetitions without an eccentric overload, performed for a single set within one minute.

Tips and Variations

Body-weight versions of the squat, hinge, and lunge can be performed for sets of 10 to 15 reps and an RPE of seven. After assessing the degree of DOMS from the arm training, horizontal pull exercises may be included with reduced volume.

Full Flex Method Execution

- The full flex method can be used on each rep. This means that you'll squeeze the active muscles hard when it is in its maximally shortened position (i.e., at the end of each concentric movement, before the eccentric movement). This doesn't need to be held for any period of time; only take as much time as necessary for you to feel maximal contraction.

SideBarr: The RPE Advantage

You might immediately see the inherent advantages of RPE-based training, because you're unable to use numerically specific loads with body-weight or elastic resistance exercises. This limitation would decrease the value of any attempt to provide traditional prescriptive programming (e.g., sets, reps, percent repetition maximum load, etc.). Consider the example of pull-ups, for which there is huge variability between individuals in their ability to execute. This means that if I were to provide a subsequent rep range, I'd have to make it as broad as 1 to 20. That range isn't guidance—it's just an attempt to prove that I can count (ostensibly using fingers *and* toes). So this application provides another example of how by using RPE, you can make the exercise as hard as you need, to personalize the resulting stimulation.

As a progression following your mastery over peak contractions, you can then stop in the middle of the eccentric rep for a maximal squeeze at this muscle length. This isometric pause is brief but incredibly challenging to do, because the muscle is lengthened compared to peak contraction. The greater the muscle length, the harder it becomes to dig in and experience the full flex. As you develop this skill, you'll be able to translate its application beyond lighter loads and ensure maximal fiber stimulation during reps with any load.

- Remember that you're not using measured weights, so your load and subsequent RPE will be regulated in real time by how much assistance you use on each rep.

- Although the rice bucket is not technically body-weight resistance, it fits perfectly with this section. Climbers, grapplers, and other body-weight training athletes are among those who experience grip and forearm improvements from this implement.

PROGRAM 2: BARE BONES BAND TRAINING

This phase uses fast concentric contractions as a novel stimulus, along with eccentric overload, to maximize growth. In the first week, you will work on getting the feel of the movements, getting used to the strength curve of the band resistance, and establishing your relative resistance (table 10.2).

You can perform these workouts with nothing more than body weight, elastic resistance, and an anchor point (pull-ups excluded). These implements are considered bare minimum, because they are widely available, inexpensive, and light. The latter translates into highly portable and useful in small spaces, like an apartment or hotel room.

The stress stimulus of time under tension induces the metabolic hypertrophy, and the eccentric overload reps cause predominantly structural growth.

The fourth week of each block is a deload period, during which the load is greatly reduced (without using any eccentric overload), or an active rest period, in which no direct strength training is performed (table 10.4, page 253).

Table 10.2 Block 1 Overview

Sets per exercise	2
Exercises per arm group	3
Tempo (TUT)	2/0/0/*
Interset rest	2-3 min

*With practice, a hard muscle squeeze in this shortened position should take less than one second.

Using soreness as a key performance indicator is especially important for exaggerated eccentric training, because you want to ensure that you are fully adapted before performing additional work on the muscle.

On the final set of each arm exercise, perform a single eccentric-overload rep (typically by stretching the band to a greater degree) using a resistance that will overload you within one or two seconds. It is natural to have to take a couple of seconds for this setup before the final rep. Increase the number of eccentric overload reps by one per exercise, each week.

BREAK-DROP-BRAKE TECHNIQUE

Band tension increases as it is stretched, so it places most of the load on the muscle at the end of the concentric ROM and the beginning of the eccentric ROM. In contrast, a greater amount of desirable microtrauma happens when there is tension on the muscle at a lengthened position (toward the end of the eccentric ROM). This limited ROM of max tension is why bands are incredible for introducing you to the novel skill of eccentric overload training—they help to minimize excessive damage and soreness that would otherwise occur with full ROM loads.

The limitation is that as you become more advanced, you're potentially limiting the amount of mechanical stress stimulus by deloading the most damaging (read: stimulating) ROM. Also, individuals who train predominantly with bands often find themselves excessively sore after they shift to gravity-based loads. This is due to the novel loading at the end ROM and can be exacerbated by momentum—neither of these variables are experienced (or adapted to) with band training.

To counter this, we'll use the **break-drop-brake technique** (aka break drop), which is inspired by the research of a strongman competitor whose physique is reminiscent of The Mountain from *Game of Thrones*, Dr. Jonathan Mike. Among the findings, Dr. Mike and his all-star research team discovered that faster eccentrics (with typical training loads; 80-85 percent 1RM) caused greater soreness compared to those that are performed more slowly (Mike et al. 2017). If we extrapolate soreness to damage in this case, the result means that we're able to trigger a massive growth stimulus—*if* we can find a safe and strategic way to increase eccentric speed.

The key words here are *safe* and *strategic*, because although there's potential to stimulate growth, haphazard application could result in injury.

To think of it in action, consider the imperceptible microcheats that many people use on every rep. After the effort of the concentric movement, it is common to briefly lose focus and subtly give up a little tension (i.e., rest) as we begin the eccentric. This instinctive break builds a little momentum, which we have to slow down as we come to the end of the ROM. In some cases, we'll even forgo a complete stop at the end. Instead, we use a little remaining momentum to help us bounce to transition from the eccentric to the concentric part of the exercise. This often goes unnoticed, but it employs a bit of our natural stretch reflex to cheat up the concentric portion.

Note that both the organic braking (disproportionately applied force toward the end of the eccentric ROM) and bounce happen when the muscle is in a lengthened position. At such longer muscle lengths, we're more susceptible to damage, which is something that we can take advantage of for maximal growth.

Also note that potential muscle-related injury is likely highest during this same lengthened ROM, which is one reason why this break drop technique is not recommended for standard resistance training. This method requires experience and control in order to be employed safely. Unfortunately, our natural tendency to focus on load quantity over stimulation quality makes the prospective use of unskilled, fast eccentric movements a recipe for disaster.

After the concentric movement and any prospective isometric contraction, begin the eccentric movement with minimal resistance for the first 50 percent of the ROM. Your goal is to then use only the remaining ROM to fully stop the load at the end of the eccentric part of the exercise.

This is best exemplified by a push-up, in which you drop to the floor from full extension. Instinctively, you'll brake the movement before you break your face, coming to a full stop at the bottom. Other body-weight exercises, such as the pull-up and Nilsson curl, are not ideally suited for this technique because we are likely to place excessive load on the shoulders. Ripping your humerus out of the glenoid fossa (aka shoulder socket) is contraindicated, so rather than using a full drop, only a slightly faster eccentric movement is performed for these exercises. Also, rather than stopping at the end of the eccentric ROM, your goal is to stop just before this point.

Recall that loaded stretching might feel good in the moment but is contraindicated, which means that you're not trying to drop into a stretch. Because of the advanced nature of this technique, only use break drops when you have the ability to perform at least 12 consecutive full ROM reps of an exercise.

When you are able to perform 12 consecutive reps on pull-ups or push-ups (both are at the end of arm day 2), replace their respective eccentric overload reps with break drop reps.

Block 2 (tables 10.3 and 10.4) maintains similar TUT but allows for a faster eccentric portion of the rep and longer isometric hold (i.e., for a whole second). An eccentric overload rep is performed on the final two sets of each arm exercise, adding one rep per set each week. By week 7 you will be performing six eccentric overload reps per exercise (2 sets × 3 reps).

Table 10.3 Block 2 Overview

Sets per exercise	2
Exercises per arm group	3
Tempo (TUT)	1/0/0/1
Interset rest	2-3 min

This four-day training program employs more intense arm-focused days and lighter whole-body days. For simplicity, the training week has been shown using seven days (table 10.5). For your applied programming, the training week is more accurately described as a microcycle, because its length consists of two arm workouts (Arms 1 and Arms 2), not necessarily a seven-day week. Stated differently, your microcycle (aka training week) is predicated on completing the requisite workouts, irrespective of time. This means, for example, if you overdo your Arms 1 session on Monday (day 1) and DOMS prevents you from executing Arms 2 until the next Monday (day 8), this still counts as a microcycle 1 workout. For this example, if you're ready to crush the Arms 1 workout on the second Thursday (11 days after you began), this will count as the start of the second microcycle (aka week 2).

Table 10.4 Summary of Bare Bones Band Training Programming Elements

Mesocycle								
Block	1				2			
Microcycle or week	1	2	3	4	5	6	7	8
Reps per set	10	8	6	Deload	8	6	4	Deload
Eccentric overload reps	1	2	3	0	2	4	6	0
RPE	6-7	7-8	8	Deload	6-7	7-8	8	Deload

Table 10.5 Microcycle Using a Seven-Day Training Week

Monday	Tuesday	Wednesday	Thursday	Friday	Saturday	Sunday
Arms 1	Body 1	Off or recovery work	Arms 2	Body 2	Off or recovery work	Off or recovery work
Standing curl (p. 148)	RDL (p. 60)		Caulfield curl (p. 132)	Bulgarian split squat (p. 66)		
Push-down (p. 112)	Suspension high row (p. 74)		Supinated extension (p. 102)	Suspension high-elbow row (p. 74)		
Spider curl (standing) (p. 134)	Reverse lunge (p. 64)		Incline curl (p. 152)	Quad-focused squat (p. 56)		
Seated 1-arm overhead extension (p. 96)	1-arm fly (p. 70)		Cross face extension (p. 104)	KB press (p. 72)		
Crush curl (p. 166)	1-arm row (p. 76)		Eccentric pull-up (p. 78)	Accessory		
Pit stain press (p. 98)	Goblet squat (p. 54)		Banded push-up (p. 94)			

Tips and Variations

- Banded variations are performed with the anchor point set to allow for tension throughout the movement that is similar to the gravity-based version. For example, the spider curl is normally executed face down on a bench with dumbbells. The adapted version uses a band anchored at shoulder height, and the movement is performed standing while facing the rack with arms straight out in front of you (i.e., parallel to the ground) throughout. Similarly, an incline curl is mimicked by facing away from the band attachment, so that your arms are behind you at the start of the movement. An adapted goblet squat anchors the band low and the other end is held in clasped hands, while you perform the squat facing away from the anchor.

- Eccentric pull-up progressions are well suited to this phase and can even serve as an effective stimulus for arm musculature. The concentric load should be light enough to allow for a rapid contraction, while the eccentric load is maintained for the suggested duration.

- The end of the fourth training day can be used for accessory work, such as abs, calves, or rice bucket training.

- To decrease the risk of excessive soreness resulting from eccentric overload reps, fatigue from the preceding set is strategically used to limit the amount of eccentric tension you use. This self-imposed throttle progressively decreases in magnitude, which allows more eccentric tension to be applied each week.

WRAP-UP

It's usually easier to achieve metabolic stimulation with limited-equipment training because body-weight–based movements can be deloaded and used for high TUT sets. It can more challenging to induce structural growth, which is why we've emphasized eccentric reps in this section, most often via resistance band overload.

To help you accomplish your arm training goals, we've covered two common types of bare bones training: body weight and banded (aka elastic resistance). A common thread that runs through their programming and descriptions is an exaggerated eccentric emphasis. Additionally, you've seen two new techniques that will help you to take advantage of each opportunity: the full flex method and the break drop.

Advanced Programming

Developing mastery of physique is analogous to becoming a master physicist. You don't learn physics more quicky by starting with an advanced field like quantum electrodynamics. In fact, doing so would probably hurt your progress. Although it may feel counterintuitive, the fastest way to reach your goal is to start with the fundamentals and progress consistently. So, once you've established the basics like bracing, tension, locus of focus, and so on, you may need to implement advanced programming for continued growth or fat loss. This should always come with a warning, because the term *advanced* can be erroneously interpreted as somehow better, just as the word *novice* may be seen as a pejorative.

Like so many others, I've experienced this mistake in practice by jumping into the very high-volume training programs of elite bodybuilders, thinking that this was the secret to faster growth. It would have been great to take advantage of the early days when just thinking about the gym could stimulate muscle, but I got caught up in the more-is-better mentality. As a result of having confused advanced training with faster gains, nearly everyone I know has started out by lifting excessively and ended up frustrated, burned out, or even injured.

In order to prevent others from repeating this mistake, each type of programming in this book considers the specific needs of the person reading it, as evidenced by the repeated importance of personalization. So, with this in mind, we'll explore advanced programs for

1. strength-based growth and
2. fat loss training.

STRENGTH AND MUSCLE

This program is not offered as a privilege that has to be earned, but rather an evolution that comes out of necessity. Consider that as muscle adapts, it becomes more resistant to the stresses we impose on it. As a consequence, we have to find new methods of stimulating hypertrophy (i.e. the principle of progression). One answer is the inclusion of heavier strength-focused training.

This more advanced program builds off of the physical foundation established by higher rep hypertrophy phases, during which tendons and ligaments become stronger and help to prepare you for heavier loads. Additional experiences with bracing, breathing, eccentrics, and reps in reserve (RIR) will all contribute to your success during this type of program.

Although this is hypertrophy-focused training, the training split is divided into three days: hypertrophy, whole body, and strength. The hypertrophy day uses higher time under tension (TUT) work used to target metabolic growth, albeit at a lower relative effort (higher RPE training is saved for strength days). (See table 11.1.) Now that you're more advanced, eccentric work will be used with greater effectiveness and less resulting soreness. This is especially true for kinetically accommodating resistance used on each hypertrophy day in this sample program.

Whole-body days employ exercises from the six foundational movements as a temporary maintenance while you focus on advanced arm training. You'll choose an exercise to represent each of the movements (except for the carry, which is covered by recovery days) and perform them for two to three sets at a moderate (~70%) relative intensity.

Strength days are the focus for your intensity during this advanced program. There are three main reasons why heavier strength training augments your hypertrophy-specific training: structural hypertrophy, strength base, and psychological adaptation.

Structural Hypertrophy

We'll apply key 4 (precision microtargeting) via heavy strength training, because it attacks the component of growth known as **structural hypertrophy** (also known as **myofibrillar hypertrophy**). The resulting stimulus causes muscle to become more resistant to the stresses of heavy loading and damage.

Table 11.1 Advanced Strength-Based Hypertrophy Overview

Sets per exercise	3
Hypertrophy day	
Tempo (TUT)	2/0/1/0
Interset rest	2 min
Strength day	
Tempo (TUT)	1/0/1/0
Interset rest	3 min

Strength Base

Moving heavier loads comes with the extrapolated benefit of being able to apply the strength you develop in this program to subsequent hypertrophy training. This means that by getting stronger overall, you'll be able to use heavier loads to generate a greater stimulus with higher rep hypertrophy training. Whether it's from the increased confidence you gain by overcoming

SideBarr: Reconsidering Repetition Maximums

We're delving into strength, which means that the concept of how much you can lift often comes into play. In order to stay on target, let's reverse engineer the concept and its application. It's common to think of a one-repetition maximum (1RM) as the maximum amount of weight you can lift, but we can upgrade this older definition to improve its fidelity and make it more consistent with anatomically targeted training (key 1). As we saw in chapter 1, the more advanced version considers the type of resistance, both types of contractions, and the full ROM. In doing so the concentric constraint and con-ROM become damning, because they expose the 1RM as merely

The maximum weight that can be overcome (1) during the weakest part of the ROM, (2) of our weakest contraction, and (3) using a gravity-based load.

In using this definition, it sounds as though traditional strength training is more appropriately identified as weakness training. Restricting your stimulus to a small part of a range of motion of one type of contraction, while simply picking up and putting down heavy stuff, really spells out how much opportunity we have for improvement. In fact, it's hard to think of other ideas that have evolved less over the past century. This is why we've focused on the concept of stress stimulus (exemplified by key 3, adaptive targeting) in this book to optimize your gains.

If your fundamental goal is to induces stresses on muscle that stimulate it to grow, the high-fidelity definition of a 1RM has exposed the emperor for having no clothes. The physical, and apparently cognitive, limits imposed by these traditional reps explains why the use of prescriptive 1RM-based loads are often constraints for your training. This doesn't mean that Iron Age 1RMs and their prescriptive use are bad or that they can't be helpful. It simply means that this gold standard has evolved. You now have better, more personalized tools to fit the job of stimulating muscle and evaluating progress—your key performance indicators (KPIs; further discussed in the Fat Loss KPIs section later in the chapter).

heavier weights or by causing a new type of central nervous system adaptation, this strength leads to long-term growth.

Psychological Adaptation

Mixing up the rep ranges, loads, and rest periods can be incredibly refreshing for anyone. Additional motivation comes from the rapid strength adaptations that you'll experience as you add weight to the bar each week. There's something incredibly empowering about this—it just feels good to be strong!

GET THE MOST OUT OF HYPERTROPHY DAYS

It may seem unusual for a hypertrophy training day to take a backseat to anything during a growth-centric program, but the following tips will help you iron out the kinks and push toward the goal of maximizing muscle size.

- The training intensity is decreased, which allows you to emphasize the strength day. The number of work sets can be increased or decreased according to your experience-based KPIs.
- Forearm work is incorporated at the end of the workout. Along with highly visible hypertrophy, increasing your grip strength will also help with strength days.
- Whole-body days are used for the six foundational movement patterns, without inducing fatigue that would impair your upcoming strength workout. This infrequent training is considered to be a temporary maintenance phase for these movements, while you focus on arm development.
- If you accidentally overdo it your hypertrophy day, the following day would be ideal for recovery work.
- On the second four-week block, replace the first two exercises (Clayton curl and JM press) with drag curls and decline dumbbell extensions. This will provide your joints some extra time to adapt.
- Block 2 also adds eccentric reps to finish off each exercise, other than pin press and forearm work (which are optional). These reps can be performed as a cluster, completed within one minute after the final concentric phase. This will add a progressive, challenging stimulus but should not cause excessive delayed-onset muscle soreness (DOMS).
- Conclude the final set of each block 2 arm-focused exercise (indicated by an asterisk in table 11.2) by adding 20 percent weight and performing a single, four-second eccentric movement. This is a bonus stimulus that does not count toward your rep total. Progress by adding an additional 10 percent per week to these reps, so that your final reps during week 9 are 50 percent heavier than your working load. This will briefly increase your relative effort, and the weights will feel heavier due to fatigue, but they won't feel heavy compared to your strength days. Note that your

perception of *heavy* will have changed after only one block of strength-based training.

- In block 1, the treadmill press is consistently performed at 50 percent of maximal effort, but it is progressed by increasing the weekly volume. This will help you get used to this unusual, but potent resistance. Begin week 1 with a cluster set of six reps per arm *total*, performed with five seconds rest between each. Progressively add one cluster of six reps per week according to your KPIs, up to a maximum of 24 reps per arm.

- In block 2, the intensity of the treadmill press will increase each week. This will help rewire your nervous system by tapping into more of your force potential. Perform two cluster sets of eight reps per arm, resting as much time as needed between reps. Your intensity will start at 60 percent, progressing 10 percent per week up to 90 percent by week 9.

GET THE MOST OUT OF STRENGTH DAYS

Even if you're pushing hard on each rep, it will probably feel as though you're not doing much to stimulate growth on these days. This is especially true when you become used to the pump and burn associated with higher rep (i.e., higher TUT) sets. Short-duration sets and long rest periods are hallmarks of maximal strength straining, which is not only something you'll get used to but something you'll actually come to appreciate. The goal of this program is still hypertrophy training, but for these blocks, you'll put your greater intensity into the strength days (see tables 11.2-4). Keep in mind the following points:

- Your sets are brief, so make them count.

- Use an external locus of focus in which you're trying to move the implement. Not only will this help you move more weight, but it's also a refreshing switch from using muscle contraction to move the load.

- The combination of brief sets and long duration between means that rest periods will feel like an eternity. To maintain efficiency (and sanity), you can perform alternating sets with exercises for each muscle group (just as you might with any hypertrophy day). Paired exercises are shown below within the same cell, and rest will be two minutes between them. For example, you can begin with your first set of barbell curls followed two minutes later by a set of bench presses. After another 120 seconds of rest, the next set of biceps curls is executed. There's nothing magical about two minutes, so rest as long as you need to crush the next set.

- You want to be as fresh as possible for each set. Unlike sets with higher TUT, fatigue is your enemy here.

- As the loads become heavier and slow down the movement of each rep, you can try to accelerate the weight for better muscle recruitment. Recall from chapter 2 that muscle recruitment is increased by the *intent* to contract quickly. Your goal is to stimulate the muscle and nervous system, so ignore the instinct to use this tip as an excuse to employ momentum as a cheat.

• Bracing and generating internal tension have great synergy with strength training. Even though you're fighting heavier loads, it might feel easier to brace because of the short set duration.

Table 11.2 Advanced Strength-Based Hypertrophy Blocks 1 and 2 Overview

Mesocycle	Advanced strength-based hypertrophy									
Block	Block 1					Block 2				
Microcycle or week	1	2	3	4	5	6	7	8	9	10
Reps (hypertrophy; strength)	12; 6	10; 5	8; 3	8; 3	Deload	12*; 5	10*; 5	8*; 3	8*; 3	Off
Relative intensity (hypertrophy; strength)	70	70; 80	70; 80	80; 90	Deload	70	70; 80	80	80; 90	Off

*Add 20 percent to your weight and perform a single, four-second eccentric movement.

Table 11.3 Advanced Strength-Based Hypertrophy Block 1 Week Overview

Monday	Tuesday	Wednesday	Thursday	Friday	Saturday	Sunday
Hypertrophy day	Rest or active recovery	Whole body	Rest or active recovery	Strength day	Rest or active recovery	Rest or active recovery
Clayton curl (p. 138)				Barbell curl (p. 148) and bench press (p. 88)		
JM press (p. 114)						
Harski hammer curl (p. 144)				Concentration curl (p. 142) and overhead rope extension (p. 108)		
Pin press (p. 110)						
X-body hammer curl (p. 164)				Cable hammer curl (p. 162) and cable push-down (p. 112)		
Treadmill press (p. 190)						
Behind-the-back wrist curl (p. 168)				Flexy bar bench (p. 196)		
Wenning wrist flicks (p. 170)						

- Maximize stability as much as possible. You don't have a ton of options here, so just remember that the fewer joints that you have to worry about stabilizing, the better. This is why concentration curls are exceptional, even though they seem like the perfect antithesis of strength-based training; the entire shoulder is supported during this exercise so you can focus on moving the load.

- As a general follow-up to the previous point: when evaluating *why* you're doing something, always come back to the rationale of your fundamental goal, rather than tradition and witchcraft.

- The overhead rope extension can be awkward to set up and perform with heavy loads. If it becomes too unwieldy, sets can be performed unilaterally (with one arm), with the resting arm serving as overhead support for the working arm.

- You're using relatively heavy loads, but you should not experience significant DOMS in your arm muscles. Your KPI for this day is discussed in detail in the next section.

- The flexy bar bench press is a great example of light accessory work that can be done to end a strength workout. It adds to your bullet proofing without detracting from your results.

Table 11.4 Advanced Strength-Based Hypertrophy Block 2 Week Overview

Monday	Tuesday	Wednesday	Thursday	Friday	Saturday	Sunday
Hypertrophy day	Rest or active recovery	Whole body	Rest or active recovery	Strength day	Rest or active recovery	Rest or active recovery
Drag curl* (p. 150)				Barbell curl (p. 148) and bench press (p. 88)		
Decline dumbbell extension* (p. 92)						
Harski hammer curl* (p. 144)				Concentration curl (p. 142) and overhead rope extension (p. 108)		
Pin press* (p. 110)						
X-body hammer curl* (p. 164)				Cable hammer curl (p. 162) and cable push-down (p. 112)		
Treadmill press (p. 190)						
Behind-the-back wrist curl (p. 168)				Flexy bar bench (p. 196)		
Wenning wrist flicks (p. 170)						

*Perform an additional eccentric rep at the end of the final set.

STRENGTH AS A KPI

Intuitively, you'll want to start each new workout in search of additional five-pound (2.3 kg) plates to throw on the bar, but this is only part of the story. While it's possible that your training loads will increase with every strength workout, your adaptations might not start off in such an obvious manner. Because a strength-focused workout can be such a contrast from traditional high TUT training, it might take you a couple of weeks just to get the right weights on the bar. So don't worry if you're not seeing overt signs right away, because the changes may be more subtle and the gains will come.

Even if you're not bumping the load each workout, you should still experience a progressive increase in perceived comfort with handling heavier loads. Also, the movements should progressively feel smoother and your overall stability much greater. If you're not feeling these changes by the end of the third strength-based workout (week 3), it's time to take a layoff (i.e., skip week 4) and evaluate.

If this happens and you can rule out lifestyle factors (e.g., nutrition, sleep, etc.), there are three likely reasons for your lack of progress. The first two default to too much work and insufficient recovery adaptation, which you may experience as general prolonged fatigue, lack of desire to train, or mood disturbances. A mood profile assessment may help you to identify this. Whatever the cause, once you've identified the general problem (i.e., lack of adaptation), you'll evaluate and adjust, using the heuristics that follow.

Prospective Cause 1: Excessive Hypertrophy Work

If you've added sets to your hypertrophy day, roll back to a reduced volume. Similarly, if you're experiencing excessive DOMS after the hypertrophy day, decrease the number of reps by 50 percent on your eccentric work.

Prospective Cause 2: Excessive Strength Work

Early strength-based training should not be taking a toll on you physically, but if it is, you need to back off the volume for the affected areas (e.g., excessive triceps DOMS). A more likely scenario is CNS burnout, in which case you will decrease intensity (based on your rating of perceived exertion) by 10 percent during phase 2.

Note that even just taking a week off could resolve the problem, allowing you to jump back in feeling stronger than ever. If this happens, consider taking more frequent breaks from training and incorporating deload weeks.

It's counterintuitive to train less and gain more, but listen to your body and experience the results. This is what personalization is all about.

Prospective Cause 3: Insufficient Strength Work

If you're not getting stronger but not experiencing any of the common symptoms associated with excessive training, you will actually need to add volume to your strength workouts. Begin with one additional set per strength exercise and reevaluate after two weeks. Note that as you add sets, your postworkout fatigue will increase. Compensate by decreasing the intensity of your hypertrophy day by 10 percent.

Note that a lack of hypertrophy work is not a factor with regard to the KPI of strength increases.

FAT LOSS TRAINING

Even for the most zealous of growth-centric lifters, there will come a time when fat loss is the goal. After all, there's no point in having great arms is all your hard work is covered up. We'll explore the advanced programming for fat loss, but unlike muscle growth, torching body fat has no direct stimulus. Instead, a general increase in energy expenditure versus consumption must be achieved through exercise and diet. Although an entire book could be written about fat loss nutrition*, we'll touch on the important basics here.

Fundamentally, the main concept of fat loss is as simple as burning more energy, in the form of calories, than is consumed. The body then taps into existing energy stores (e.g., body fat) to maintain energy needs during this caloric deficit. The challenge happens because your body perceives this controlled starvation as a threat to survival and wants to respond by getting rid of your most metabolically active (read: energy consuming) tissue. Unfortunately, this energy-burning tissue is your hard-earned muscle. Its loss is a double negative, because less muscle means less muscularity, *and* less 24-hour fat burning. The great news is that there are two main ways to mitigate this breakdown: resistance training and protein intake.

Resistance Training

It may seem exceedingly obvious considering where you're reading this, but think about how many people go on a diet (i.e., induce a caloric deficit in an attempt to lose body fat) at some point in their life. Of these, what is the miniscule percentage of those who lift throughout this period of caloric restriction? Because you are one of those few, you're already ahead of the game.

---

* *See the SideBarr on the next page.*

SideBarr

If you're looking for a science-based source of nutrition information, I recommend checking out *NSCA's Guide to Sport and Exercise Nutrition, Second Edition* (Human Kinetics, 2021). I authored the Protein chapter and, yes, am horribly (*horribly*) biased.

Protein Intake

Although you're dropping calories from nutrient sources (carbs and fats), you'll want to maintain or possibly even increase your protein intake. This will help to preserve the metabolic machine that is your muscle. Impactful evidence of this came from the lab of one of my research mentors, Dr. Kevin Tipton (Mettler, Mitchell, and Tipton 2010). The team found that among resistance-trained athletes who underwent two weeks of caloric restriction, more lean body mass was retained in a group that consumed 2.3 g of protein/kg body weight compared to those who ingested 1 g protein/kg body weight daily.

Zombie Cardio

There's a lot of miscommunication about cardiovascular activity and fat burning. Most fundamentally, this comes with the Iron Age idea that resistance training builds muscle, while cardio burns fat. This zombie myth needs to be stabbed in the brain and then torched along with your body fat.

Although cardio is a great secondary training method to burn calories, resistance training is the priority. Recall that your goal is to preserve (or even build) muscle and stimulate energy expenditure over the course of each 24-hour day. Traditional low-intensity cardio might burn a greater proportion of fat for energy while you're doing it, but the overall energy expenditure is limited. This means less of a caloric deficit and therefore less fat loss over 24 hours.

Additionally, it's important to know that the fat you burn can come from different sources, like your blood or muscle stores, not necessarily the adipose tissue covering your abs. This doesn't make cardio bad; it just means that the hype of cardio and any associated short-term fat burning is overblown. Ideally, we want to find a way to make low intensity exercise work better for you, which goes beyond calories or a transient fat-burning zone. It begins by exploring your body's metabolic machinery, which you can then upgrade through a strategic combination of training and nutrition.

Metabolic Flexibility

Your body has two main energy sources, one fast and one slow. Carbs are an inefficient, but quickly available source, which provide most of the energy during lifts, for example. When you're not performing high-intensity exercise, your body can rely on internal fat stores to meet energy demands. Fats are the most efficient energy source, which is why you're using them for energy right now, but it takes a long time for this delivery system to ramp up when demands increase (e.g., during exercise).

Based on the demand, your body will shift back and forth between these sources. For example, whenever fat burning is insufficient to provide adequate energy, your body shifts to carb burning. This is important to know when you have a goal of decreasing body fat, because you'll want to make it easier for your body to shift into a fat-burning state. This concept, called **metabolic flexibility (met flex)**, was introduced to me by Dr. Mike T. Nelson, associate professor at the Carrick Institute. He explains it in the following way, "Metabolic flexibility refers to your body's ability to shift between the use of fat and carbs for energy. The more metabolically flexible you are, the better your performance and fat loss" (Mike T. Nelson, pers. comm).

Along with your diet and resistance training, adding lower intensity activity might help teach your body to burn fat. The simplest way to do this is to ensure that you consume relatively more carbs for your lift, which will allow you to have a better workout and greater muscle stimulus. To facilitate a shift toward fat utilization, your lower intensity exercise occurs after a period of relatively lower carb intake.

In contrast to the zombie myth discussed earlier, you're not worried about the immediate effect of fat use during this exercise. You're using this strategy for its potential to improve your long-term ability to use fat for energy (i.e., increase your met flex). The combination of maintaining muscle and a net caloric expenditure, along with a greater proportion of that energy coming from fat, will have you showing off triceps striations in no time.

SideBarr

If it seems like your muscles are deflating during this period, remember from chapter 8 (Recovery Optimization) that your muscles are filled with glycogen and water. Burning through the stored carbs and losing some of the accompanying water will naturally decrease muscle size until you replenish those glycogen stores (via higher caloric or carb intake).

Strategy 1: More Calories Burned

- Increased caloric expenditure through muscle maintenance and growth
- Prioritized resistance training
- Increased relative protein intake

Strategy 2: Greater Proportion of Calories Burned From Fat

- Improved met flex to increase the contribution of fat-derived calories
- Low-intensity, low-impact sustained exercise

LOW-INTENSITY EXERCISE

As you begin to use a higher training volume, be aware that your low-intensity exercise (also known as cardio) has the potential to interfere with your resistance training. To mitigate this possibility, your low-intensity training should be low impact and eccentric exercise free. This means that you're better off using traditional cardio machines like a cycle ergometer or elliptical machine, instead of running (for example). Better yet, we've covered another great tool for the job in previous chapters—sled work. This provides resistance in the horizontal plane, in contrast to the gravity-based vertical loading you get from loaded carries or running. Considering the large amount of training volume on your legs during this program, you want to minimize further vertical loading.

You can use the arm-focused movements discussed earlier, but you'll predominantly use consistent pace walking, either pushing on the sled or pulling it by walking away. During this sustained sled work, you'll maintain consistent tension on the connector as you walk against the resistance of the load (unlike repetition-based sled work).

FAT LOSS KPIS

The fat loss program is considered to be advanced, because it builds off of the principles that you've honed through practice, such as locus of focus. This will ensure that you can stimulate the muscle to a greater degree, which helps to achieve the results you're after. Additionally, you'll have had practice with the anatomically targeted exercises, which gives you a background of your personalized KPIs. Armed with this knowledge, you can track relative changes in your strength along with how quickly you fatigue during a set.

You should be able to maintain your strength and RIR estimates with this program, and slight changes in these KPIs are nothing to worry about (especially as you feel your way through the new diet). What you want to watch for are abrupt changes in strength or RIR. Although it could just reflect an off day, if it happens in consecutive workouts, you'll want to respond by evaluating your diet and training.

Although the adjustment will take the form of increased calories or reduced training load, we don't want to go too far beyond the wide-ranging examples in the list that follows. Note that the breadth of these changes also serves to illustrate why this is an advanced program: there are a lot of considerations and components to evaluate and potentially adjust. Generalized examples of prospective changes include the following:

- Increased carb intake in the hours before your lift
- Increased daily protein intake
- Decreased volume of low-intensity exercise
- Taking a day or two off from training
- Stopping the caloric restriction altogether

When using a calorie-restricted diet simply to look better, rather than for health reasons, it's important to know that you can stop it at any time, for any reason. Fat loss won't come without sacrifice, but there's no need to agonize. *The most effective fat loss diet is the one that you can stick with.* So if you're just not into it this time around, stop and reset.

Among the many preventable issues you've seen to achieve successful long-term fat loss, the final upgrade happens when you increase calorie consumption to prestarvation levels. Although traditional thinking is that one can go on a diet to lose body fat, only to return to the same prediet conditions that increased adiposity in the first place, this, combined with changes in scale weight, is what contributes to yo-yo dieting. The greatest success happens when you continually make small incremental changes to your lifestyle, engrain these changes as habits, and celebrate the accomplishment of each progressive upgrade.

As a personalized gauge of exercise intensity, you will use the **progressive talk test**. This means that you want to exert the maximal amount of effort that will enable you to speak normally (without excessive panting). The progressive element considers the slow ramp-up of fat metabolism that happens during this type of exercise. Throughout each low-intensity workout (starting from minute 1), you'll continually provide more and more of your energy needs with fat. This natural shifting toward high-yield fat metabolism means that you'll be able to gradually increase intensity within each session. As you become more metabolically flexible over the long term, you'll notice this shift happen earlier and to a greater degree.

This program is a modified version of the four-day program from chapter 9 (table 9.4). The main difference is the inclusion of two low-intensity days. The duration (in minutes) of these sessions is indicated in tables 11.5-7.

Table 11.5 Advanced Fat Loss Training Overview

Sets per exercise	3
Exercises per arm group	3
Tempo (TUT)	2/0/1/0
Interset rest	2 min

Table 11.6 Advanced Fat Loss Blocks 1 and 2 Overview

Mesocycle	Advanced fat loss									
Block	Block 1					Block 2				
Microcycle or week	1	2	3	4	5	6	7	8	9	10
Reps	12	10	8	8	Deload	12	10	8	8	Off
RIR	3	2	1	0	Deload	3	2	1	0	Off
Low-intensity duration	40	50	60	60	30	60	60	60	60	Off

Table 11.7 Advanced Fat Loss Block 1 Week Overview

Monday	Tuesday	Wednesday	Thursday	Friday	Saturday	Sunday
Biceps day 1	**Triceps day 1**	**Low intensity sustained**	**Biceps day 2**	**Triceps day 2**	**Low intensity sustained**	**Off**
Barbell curl (p. 148)	Bench press (p. 88)		Preacher curl (p. 130)	Banded push-up (p. 94)		
Reverse lunge (p. 64)	Suspension high row (p. 74)		Bulgarian split squat (p. 66)	Pull-down, pull-up (p. 78)		
Cable flex curl (p. 146)	Seated overhead dumbbell extension (p. 96)		Incline dumbbell curl (p. 152)	Overhead rope extension (p. 108)		
Cable fly (p. 70)	Goblet squat (p. 54)		Kettlebell press (p. 72)	Quad-focused squat (p. 56)		
X-body hammer curl (p. 164)	Pit stain press (p. 98)		Pronated barbell curl (p. 161)	Supinated cable extension (p. 102)		
Ball hamstring curl (p. 62)			Suitcase carry (p. 80)			

WRAP-UP

This ultimate chapter builds on your preexisting physical preparation and highlights advanced methods of strength-based growth and training for fat loss. The use of strength for growth may seem contradictory at first but can be a great fit once you've established solid physical condition through the application of earlier chapters. Even if you're not fat-focused yet, there will come a time when you are. Once again, the associated advanced program will help you to chisel your physique from the rock-solid foundation developed through earlier chapters.

Ultimate SideBarr

Although this book is the result of nearly three decades of obsession, education, and experimentation, the greatest innovation comes from the dozens of would-be contributors who have taught me along the way. As that brilliant torch is passed, it is worth offering one final Side-Barr. Reminiscent of early primates running from their first glimpse of a cooking fire, innovation is often met with fear and contempt. It takes time for the parasite of our own psychology to extract itself from the comfort of tradition and seems to inflict unnecessary pain while doing so. But rather than a gradual transition into acceptance, we tend to erect a cognitive partition that grants us amnesia for our having ever resisted those ideas. Instead, the once-derided novelty suddenly becomes all too obvious for us. Like flipping a switch, the initial sentiments of "That idea is stupid!" are quickly replaced with the clarity of "*Everyone* knows that!" In doing so, we skip out on the best part, which is the excitement generated by an idea that is both new and useful.

This "fear to clear" switch is a psychological phenomenon that affects all of us, and it is aligned with this book's recurring theme of opportunity. By becoming aware of our primitive resistance to change we're better equipped to overcome it. This allows us to hit the sweet spot and become motivated to apply novel strategies in our ongoing hunt for personal development. So, rather than running from the fire, we become illuminated by it. If nothing else, this light will help you to show off your new set of massive, muscular arms.

Until next time, Raise The Barr!

Glossary

accommodating resistance—Change in the force of resistance throughout the ROM of exercise, as a result of your action against it.

adaptation—Going beyond where you started. This is where you get bigger, faster, and stronger. Ultimately, this is what you're after.

adaptive recovery—Type of technique that works with the body's natural biochemistry to facilitate recovery adaptation.

anabolic—Characterized by the process of building muscle.

anchoring—The process of standardizing intensity across individuals.

antagonist muscles—Those muscles that perform opposing actions, like the biceps and triceps.

autoregulation—The use of personal feedback to adjust your training to your abilities on that day.

biceps muscle—The large arm muscle between the shoulder and forearm that we associate with the biceps and triceps muscles.

blue shifting—Decreasing recovery time and time to peak adaptation (i.e., they are happening faster), indicated by a shortened wavelength on the recovery adaptation curve. This is consistent with blunting (also known as decreasing) the adaptive response.

brachialis—An elbow flexor muscle that lies beneath the biceps.

brachioradialis—An elbow flexor muscle that is highly visible on the forearm.

bracing—Establishing stabilizing tension throughout your core.

brand annihilation—When a specific brand name is used to represent an entire product category.

break-drop-brake technique—Disproportionately applied force toward the end of the eccentric ROM. This is done to increase the eccentric stress stimulus from otherwise light loads. Also known as break drops.

carrying angle—The angle created at your elbow by the difference in alignment between your arm and forearm.

casein—A slow-digesting, milk-derived protein. This protein clots in the stomach and is slowly digested to provide a steady trickle of amino acids to the body.

catabolic—Characterized by the process of muscle breakdown.

central nervous system (CNS)—*See* nervous system.

cluster training—Sets during which a brief rest (e.g., a few seconds) is taken after each rep.

concentric constraint (con-con)—Concept that illustrates the fact that we immediately limit the load of every training set based on our weakness of the concentric portion of the rep.

concentric contractions—The shortening of a muscle by producing more force than that which is opposing it.

con-ROM (concentric range of motion)—The portion of the full concentric ROM that requires the greatest force output (also known as the sticking point). This is the weakest part of the rep, which subsequently establishes the 1RM load.

consecutive contraction limit—A further reduced training load (from the con-ROM) necessary to perform consecutive full ROM contractions, which we know as a set. Typically expressed as a percent of 1RM, and often used for Iron Age prescriptive programming.

creatine monohydrate—A supplement with decades of published research supporting its efficacy and safety. Technically, it is a water molecule attached to that of creatine.

creatine—A fast-acting energy source that exists within every cell of the human body.

destructive recovery—Recovery intervention that destroys the stress response, thereby sacrificing adaptation, in order to minimize recovery time.

eccentric contraction—Active lengthening of the muscle (also known as negative) that happens when the opposing force is greater than that exerted by the muscle. This is not to be confused with muscle relaxation.

eccentric paradox—The fact that we are stronger eccentrically but produce less force during this part of the contraction. This extends the force deficit in both directions. Also known as the bidirectional eccentric paradox.

external locus of focus—The attention on moving the load.

extreme force delta—The potential for an exercise to be completely deloaded at some point of its natural ROM.

feeder workouts—Workouts using a combination of the following elements to facilitate recovery adaptation: nutrition, contraction, and sympathetic shifting.

fight or flight—A term exemplifying an excited or sympathetic state of arousal.

flexion—A movement that decreases the angle between two body parts.

force deficit—The difference between your force potential and actual forces produced during training.

force delta—The difference between the minimum and maximum required force production across an exercise ROM.

force potential—The maximum force one is capable of producing during an exercise.

force-accommodating resistance—Resistance (exerted against you) in which the force changes based on the amount of force you're exerting. Also known as tonically accommodating resistance.

forced eccentric movement—Movement made while attempting to perform a concentric contraction even though the muscle is forced eccentrically. Also known as an overwhelming eccentric.

foundational movement patterns—The six fundamental movements on which most exercises are based: squat, hinge, lunge, push, pull, and carry.

full flex method—Squeezing your working musculature as hard as possible to experience stronger, more precise contractions and deliver a more effective stress stimulus.

grip delta—The difference in natural grip width between the top and bottom of a biceps curl, caused by the carrying angle.

homeostasis—A physiologically balanced set point.

hypertrophy—Muscle growth.

humerus—The arm bone. Located between the shoulder and forearm.

index and thumb grip—Grip that involves resting the implement against the index finger and thumb side of your hand. Used with a neutral grip for forearm and brachioradialis recruitment.

intermediate recovery—A period that happens within the minutes and early hours after a lift.

internal locus of focus—Putting your attention into squeezing the muscle to move the load throughout the entire rep.

intraworkout—The time during the training session.

Iron Age thinking—The cognitive limits that have trapped our applied understanding of muscle stimulation within the Iron Age. These constraints tether us to the idea of overcoming gravity-based loads for exercises, sets and reps, and predictive programming.

Iron Age training—Traditional archaic methods of training and prescription, using exclusively gravity-based loads (also known as iron) and percent repetition maximums, respectively. Also known as dinosaur training.

isokinetic equipment—Computer-controlled machines that move the implement (e.g., a bar) at a predetermined speed, no matter how hard you push against them.

isometric contractions—Contractions in which the muscle does not shorten or lengthen because the forces exerted are matched with those that are opposing.

key performance indicators (KPIs)—Methods to evaluate training response and personalize subsequent training.

kinetically accommodating resistance—Resistance in which your ability to exert force (also known as strength, also known as force potential) changes as a result of the speed of contraction. The faster you are forced eccentrically, the more force you can produce.

localized muscle fatigue—A decreased ability to produce force in a specific muscle or muscle group.

locked grip—Grip in which an implement does not allow your wrist to rotate. Also known as fixed wrist.

long-term recovery—The adaptation phase during which your body begins to rebuild the damaged tissue and get back to where you started.

long-term recovery adaptation—A desired four-phase process that happens over the course of several days following your workout and ends with an adaptive response (e.g., increased muscle size). The phases include workout (phase 1, stress stimulus), your body's natural stress response (phase 2, aka the preadaptation phase), long-term recovery (phase 3), and adaptation (phase 4).

metabolic flexibility (met flex)—Your body's ability to shift between the use of fat and carbs for energy.

metabolic hypertrophy—The result of adaptations induced by training stresses that are related to short-term energy production and metabolic waste removal. Also known as sarcoplasmic hypertrophy.

mood state—One's current emotional disposition.

muscle protein synthesis—The growth, recovery, and adaptation response we seek through training.

myofibrillar hypertrophy—*See* structural hypertrophy.

nervous system—The body's rapid communication network.

nutraceutical effect—A direct biochemical change induced by consuming a food or specific nutrient source.

1-repetition maximum (1RM)—The maximum load that you can overcome (with good form) for a single repetition.

overtraining—An accumulation of training stresses resulting in long-term decrements to performance.

palmar grip—Grip on an implement at the center of the handle, so that the friction of your grip across your palm and fingers transmits the force you exert.

panda training—Training that causes excessive fatigue during instability training, such that bar control is lost (i.e., the load dumps).

parasympathetic—A state of low arousal when the body is relaxed or feeding.

percent RM (%RM)—A load based on a relative proportion of one's maximal ability to successfully complete a concentric repetition. For example, 65% of 1RM refers to 65% of the load for which a full concentric ROM can be completed a maximum of once.

personalization—The action of designing one's training to meet their individual requirements.

pinch grip—When an object is held between the palmar surface of the extended fingers and the opposing thumb.

pinky grip—Grip on an implement so that much of the force is transmitted across the pinky finger side of your hand. Used for triceps movements.

postworkout KPIs—Key performance indicators that occur following the workout.

premature acceleration—A common error that happens when the speed of an isokinetic eccentric movement is increased before the user learns how to contract maximally against an overwhelming force. The result is reduced magnitude of adaptation.

preworkout activation—Using the immediate preworkout period to physically and mentally prepare for the upcoming workout.

progression—Principle that considers how the other training variables change over the course of weeks or months.

progressive recovery—*See* adaptive recovery.

progressive talk test—A low-intensity cardiovascular activity KPI, during which one exerts the maximal amount of effort that will enable him to speak normally (without excessive panting). The progressive element considers the slow ramp-up of fat metabolism and subsequent ability to increase intensity that happens throughout this type of exercise.

pronated grip—Grip used in elbow flexion exercises performed with an overhand or neutral wrist position. Also known as a semipronated grip.

pronation—Rotation of the hand and forearm so that the palm faces down.

proportionality principle—The concept that adaptive response is proportional to that of the stress stimulus (i.e., workout).

protein pulse feeding—Periodically consuming a fast-absorbing protein (like whey) to cyclically increase and decrease amino acids in the blood. The intent is to stimulate muscle protein synthesis.

radial deviation—The movement of bending the wrist on the thumb side of the hand.

radius—The forearm bone that is lateral when the wrist is supinated.

range of motion (ROM)—The degree of movement that happens throughout an exercise, which is typically limited by the mobility of the joint.

rating of perceived exertion (RPE)—A quantification of your degree of effort using a 0 to 10 scale.

recovery—A return to where you started prior to having experienced a deficit (e.g., a return to zero).

recruit—The activation of muscle fibers.

red shifting—Lengthening recovery and adaptation times, indicated by a graphically longer wavelength on the recovery adaptation curve. This is usually associated with an adaptive response of increased magnitude (also known as bigger gains).

reps in reserve (RIR)—An estimation of how many reps you have left in the tank when you complete a set.

rest and digest—A term exemplifying a relaxed or parasympathetic state of arousal.

reverse engineering—Developing a thorough understanding of a concept by breaking it down into its component parts.

sacrificial recovery—*See* destructive recovery.

scapula—The shoulder blade.

Selye recovery adaptation curve—A sinusoidal curve used to illustrate the natural phases of long-term recovery adaptation.

shoulder lock technique—An anatomical stability method in which you brace your elbows in front of you, so they are naturally stabilized by your torso (effectively locking your arms in place).

spatially accommodating resistance—Type of resistance that occurs when the resistance changes with distance of movement (e.g., elastic bands and chains).

specificity—The design of a training program to elicit a particular adaptive response.

sticking point—The portion of the ROM that provides the greatest challenge.

stress response—Part of long-term recovery adaptation that occurs in the hours and days following the workout in order to prepare the muscle for adaptation. It is the time when your body clears away damaged tissue through the necessary process of inflammation, which you may temporarily experience as delayed-onset muscle soreness (DOMS), swelling, decreased strength, and so on.

stress stimulus—Positive stress used to stimulate long-term adaptation. Happens by overloading the muscle during your workout and starts the entire cascade.

structural hypertrophy—Adaptation that is initiated by muscle tension and damage stresses, resulting in larger and tougher muscle.

supination—Rotation of the hand and forearm so that the palm faces up.

sympathetic nervous system—An anatomical subdivision of the nervous system responsible for increased arousal.

sympathetic shifting—Moving from an excited fight or flight state to one that is more relaxed (rest and digest).

systemic fatigue—A general tiredness or lack of energy.

targeted training parameters—Exercise programming variables.

tempo—Indicator of how quickly you perform each of the four parts of a repetition: eccentric, maximal extended position, concentric, and peak contraction. Each section is numerically expressed in seconds.

time under tension (TUT)—Method that reflects how long a muscle is working under load during a set.

triceps muscle—The muscle associated with the back of the arm.

type—The kind of equipment used within a resistance training program. Examples include dumbbells, kettlebells, and medicine balls.

ulna—The forearm bone that is medial when the wrist is supinated.

ulnar deviation—The movement of bending the wrist on the pinky finger side of the hand.

unlocked grip—Grip in which an implement allows your wrist to rotate. Also known as open wrist.

wrist extensors—Muscles on the back of the forearm.

wrist flexors—Muscles on the palmar side of the forearm.

zombie myths—Those myths that refuse to die (not myths about zombies).

References

INTRODUCTION

Benito, P. J., Cupeiro, R., Ramos-Campo, D. J., Alcaraz, P. E., & Rubio-Arias, J. Á. 2020. A Systematic Review with Meta-Analysis of the Effect of Resistance Training on Whole-Body Muscle Growth in Healthy Adult Males. *International journal of environmental research and public health, 17*(4), 1285.

CHAPTER 1

Barakat C, Barroso R, Alvarez M, Rauch J, Miller N, Bou-Sliman A, De Souza EO. 2019. "The Effects of Varying Glenohumeral Joint Angle on Acute Volume Load, Muscle Activation, Swelling, and Echo-Intensity on the Biceps Brachii in Resistance-Trained Individuals." *Sports (Basel)*. Sep 4;7(9):204.

Kleiber T, Kunz L, Disselhorst-Klug C. 2015. "Muscular coordination of biceps brachii and brachioradialis in elbow flexion with respect to hand position." *Frontiers in physiology*. 6;6:215.

CHAPTER 2

American College of Sports Medicine, G. Liguori. 2021. *ACSM's Guidelines for Exercise Testing and Prescription*, 11th ed. Philadelphia: Wolters Kluwer.

Haun, C. T., Vann, C. G., Roberts, B. M., Vigotsky, A. D., Schoenfeld, B. J., & Roberts, M. D. 2019. A Critical Evaluation of the Biological Construct Skeletal Muscle Hypertrophy: Size Matters but So Does the Measurement. *Frontiers in physiology, 10*, 247.

Mattocks, K. T., Jessee, M. B., Mouser, J. G., Dankel, S. J., Buckner, S. L., Bell, Z. W., Owens, J. G., Abe, T., & Loenneke, J. P. 2018. The Application of Blood Flow Restriction: Lessons From the Laboratory. *Current sports medicine reports, 17*(4), 129–134.

Schoenfeld, B. J., Grgic, J., Haun, C., Itagaki, T., & Helms, E. R. 2019. Calculating Set-Volume for the Limb Muscles with the Performance of Multi-Joint Exercises: Implications for Resistance Training Prescription. *Sports (Basel, Switzerland), 7*(7), 177.

Soares S, Ferreira-Junior JB, Pereira MC, Cleto VA, Castanheira RP, Cadore EL, Brown LE, Gentil P, Bemben MG, Bottaro M. 2015. "Dissociated Time Course of Muscle Damage Recovery Between Single- and Multi-Joint Exercises in Highly Resistance-Trained Men." *Journal of Strength and Conditioning Research*. 29 (9): 2594-2599.

Wackerhage, H., Schoenfeld, B. J., Hamilton, D. L., Lehti, M., & Hulmi, J. J. 2019. Stimuli and sensors that initiate skeletal muscle hypertrophy following resistance exercise. *Journal of applied physiology* (Bethesda, Md. : 1985), 126(1), 30–43.

CHAPTER 3

Schoenfeld, B.J., J. Grgic, D. Ogborn, and J.W. Krieger. 2017. "Strength and Hypertrophy Adaptations Between Low- vs. High-Load Resistance Training: A Systematic Review and Meta-Analysis." *Journal of Strength and Conditioning Research* 31 (12): 3508-3523.

Schoenfeld, B.J., A Vigotsky, B. Contreras, S. Golden, A. Alto, R. Larson, N. Winkelman, and A. Paoli. 2018. "Differential Effects of Attentional Focus Strategies During Long-Term Resistance Training." *European Journal of Sport Science* 18 (5): 705-712.

CHAPTER 6

Krings, B. M., Shepherd, B. D., Swain, J. C., Turner, A. J., Chander, H., Waldman, H. S., McAllister, M. J., Knight, A. C., & Smith, J. W. (2019). Impact of Fat Grip Attachments on Muscular Strength and Neuromuscular Activation During Resistance Exercise. *Journal of strength and conditioning research*, 10.1519/JSC.0000000000002954.

CHAPTER 7

Behm, D.G., and D.G. Sale. 1993. "Intended Rather Than Actual Movement Velocity Determines Velocity-Specific Training Response." *Journal of Applied Physiology* 74 (1): 359-368.

CHAPTER 8

Barr, D. 2008. *The Anabolic Index: Optimized Nutrition and Supplementation Manual.* Montreal: Lepine Publishing, pp. 45-48.

Dziembowska, I., P. Izdebski, A. Rasmus, J. Brudny, M. Grzelczak, and P. Cysewski. 2016. "Effects of Heart Rate Variability Biofeedback on EEG Alpha Asymmetry and Anxiety Symptoms in Male Athletes: A Pilot Study." *Applied Psychophysiology and Biofeedback* 41 (2): 141-150.

Kreider, R.B., D.S. Kalman, J. Antonio, T.N. Ziegenfuss, R. Wildman, R. Collins, D.G. Candow, S.M. Kleiner, A.L. Almada, and H.L. Lopez. 2017. "International Society of Sports Nutrition Position Stand: Safety and Efficacy of Creatine Supplementation in Exercise, Sport, and Medicine." *Journal of the International Society of Sports Nutrition* 14 (June 13): 18.

Moore, D.R., J. Areta, V.G. Coffey, T. Stellingwerff, S.M. Phillips, L.M. Burke, M. Cléroux, J.P. Godin, and J.A. Hawley. 2012. "Daytime Pattern of Post-Exercise Protein Intake Affects Whole-Body Protein Turnover in Resistance-Trained Males." *Nutrition & Metabolism* 9: 91.

Sapolsky, R.M. 2004. *Why Zebras Don't Get Ulcers: A Guide to Stress, Stress Related Diseases, and Coping, 3rd ed.* New York: Holt, Henry & Company, Inc.

Shimomura, Y., Y. Yamamoto, G. Bajotto, J. Sato, T. Murakami, N. Shimomura, H. Kobayashi, and K. Mawatari. 2006. "Nutraceutical Effects of Branched-Chain Amino Acids on Skeletal Muscle." *Journal of Nutrition* 136 (2): 529S-532S.

Tiidus, P.M. 2015. "Alternative Treatments for Muscle Injury: Massage, Cryotherapy, and Hyperbaric Oxygen." *Current Reviews in Musculoskeletal Medicine* 8 (2): 162-167.

Trommelen, J., and L.J. van Loon. 2016. "Pre-Sleep Protein Ingestion to Improve the Skeletal Muscle Adaptive Response to Exercise Training." *Nutrients* 8 (12): E763.

CHAPTER 9

Helms, E.R., J. Cronin, A. Storey, and M.C. Zourdos. 2016. "Application of the Repetitions in Reserve-Based Rating of Perceived Exertion Scale for Resistance Training." *Strength & Conditioning Journal* 38 (4): 42-49.

Ormsbee, M.J., J.P. Carzoli, A. Klemp, B.R. Allman, M.C. Zourdos, J.S. Kim, and L.B. Panton. 2019. "Efficacy of the Repetitions in Reserve-Based Rating of Perceived Exertion for the Bench Press in Experienced and Novice Benchers." *The Journal of Strength and Conditioning Research* 33 (2): 337-345.

CHAPTER 10

Schoenfeld, B.J., M.D. Peterson, D. Ogborn, B. Contreras, and G.T. Sonmez. 2015. "Effects of Low- vs. High-Load Resistance Training on Muscle Strength and Hypertrophy in Well-Trained Men." *The Journal of Strength and Conditioning Research* 29 (10): 2954-2963.

Mike, J.N., N. Cole, C. Herrera, T. VanDusseldorp, L. Kravitz, and C.M. Kerksick. 2017. "The Effects of Eccentric Contraction Duration on Muscle Strength, Power Production, Vertical Jump, and Soreness." *The Journal of Strength and Conditioning Research* 31 (3): 773-786.

CHAPTER 11

Campbell, B., ed. 2020. *NSCA's Guide to Sport and Exercise Nutrition*, 2nd ed. Champaign, IL: Human Kinetics.

Mettler, S., N. Mitchell, and K.D. Tipton. 2010. "Increased Protein Intake Reduces Lean Body Mass Loss During Weight Loss in Athletes." *Medicine & Science in Sports & Exercise* 42 (2): 326-337.